BOOST
YOUR
IMMUNE
SYSTEM

How to fight infections naturally

JENNIFER MEEK

ION
PRESS

First published in 1996
by ION Press
34, Wadham Road
London SW15 2LR
Tel: 0181-871 2949
Fax: 0181-874 5003

Illustrations & cover: Christopher Quayle
and Jonathan Phillips
Layout: Heather James

ISBN 1 870976 14 5

Printed and bound in Great Britain by the Bath Press

CONTENTS

INTRODUCTION

Welcome to the wonderful world of the immune system. To help you on your journey through this book, here are some guidelines:

Part 1 helps you to see to what extent your diet, lifestyle and environment may be affecting your immune system and enables you to assess your own immune power.

Part 2 helps you to understand what the immune system is all about. It's a complex defence mechanism, but don't be put off by all the 'new words' used to describe the different kinds of immune cells and their functions. The detail is there for those who want to go into depth, otherwise a light read will give you a good understanding of how your immune system works.

Part 3 explains how being fit and having a positive frame of mind can boost your immunity, as well as how to fight colds, plus a detailed chapter on HIV.

Part 4 gives you practical information about how to achieve optimum nutrition as a means to boosting your immunity and overall health.

Have a good journey and I wish you well in putting this information into practice in your life.

Part 1

ARE YOU IMMUNE?

1

YOUR LIFE IN YOUR HANDS

In youth and sometimes in middle age, it is easy to fool yourself into believing that all of those degenerative and life threatening diseases only happen to other people. But do they? Is there anything that you could be doing to help your immune system to keep you in good health and free from disease? How can you improve your immune system and work with it to make you look better, feel better, perform better and last longer?

What is needed is a "trouble free motor guide to our human machine" but each model is different. You are unique, there is no one else quite like you. You also are constantly changing and have different requirements at different stages in life.

There are some general guidelines, however, which will help you to steer a course through life, avoiding trouble spots and maximising performance. You have the ability (within obvious limits) to change your shape, your personality, your attitude to life, your general fitness and your resistance to disease.

Your immune system is your own personal medical team, skilled in the art of healing, always on call, (though often forgotten and neglected) and always on hand to take preventative measures to avert a battle, provided you give them the ammunition and equipment to do their job properly.

Whatever body you have now, it can be better and stronger if you co-operate with this immune system. You and your body are after all, a life long partnership and there is no getting away from it. Whether trying to prevent or needing to cure an illness your immune system is your main line of defence. It is worth looking after it so that it can serve you actively and reliably, allowing you to enjoy a happy, healthy life.

Good health is rarely achieved by chance. To keep it we have to maintain a good biochemical balance. Almost all diseases can be traced back to some chemical disturbance in the body and that imbalance may be caused by any one or a combination of factors from genetic faults to environmental poisons, malnutrition, emotional conflicts or infectious agents.

Medical science has conquered many of the killer diseases we used to have, by improving hygiene standards and developing medicines such as antibiotics which destroy the bacteria responsible, or vaccines that prevent the diseases.

Incidences of heart and circulatory diseases, cancer, auto-immune and immune related diseases are increasing rapidly. Modern killer conditions are not so easy to attack as there is often not just one single cause but a group of contributory factors. It is much more difficult to identify these and to test them because there are several interrelated variables to test at the same time. In addition there have been many changes to our modern world which are partly responsible for these 'new' illnesses.

Within the passage of a few years we have changed our food, air, water and movement; in fact our whole way of living, and we expect our bodies to adapt quickly, to find new ways of disposing of or storing safely all of the new pesticides, food additives, drugs, domestic detergents and other chemicals it comes across. All new waste substances have to be detoxified within us if they are to do no harm.

Nutrients found naturally in our food are often no longer sufficient to allow our immune system to cope efficiently with the increasing problems. Ironically, at this period in history with boats, cars, trains and planes we need less food. There are a lot of overweight people whose calorie intake exceeds need but, at the same time, we need more nutrients to help us cope with the extra pollution and stress. In food manufacture and preparation, however, we are busy processing nutrients out of food and eating far too much of the nutrient deficient, empty calorie products.

There are many enemies to a happy, healthy, efficient immune system. Some are listed below. As in any war, the fewer enemies you have attacking you at any one time, the more likely you are to remain in control and win the battle. How many could you identify and eliminate or reduce? Are there any others that you need to add to your specific list perhaps as a result of your occupation or an environmental hazard?

These are some of our main enemies and we cannot avoid them all. The best we can do is to reduce as many as possible and boost our immune systems to cope with the rest.

Enemies of the Immune System

Smoke (tobacco and other - chimneys, incinerators, etc)
Stress
Pollution (busy roads, aeroplane flight path, industry, etc)
Pesticides
Radiation
Carcinogenic chemicals (industrial or domestic)
Drugs (legal, illegal, medical - all requiring medical supervision for reduction or elimination, do not try it alone)
Food additives (especially colours and flavours)
Incorrect balance of food (eg too much salt, fat or sugar).
Accidents
Obesity or starvation (including some dangerous forms of slimming/dieting)
Poor mineral balance
Poor vitamin balance
Inappropriate exercise
Genetic defect
Infections (from bacteria, viruses, fungi, protozoa, worms, etc.)
Negative attitudes to life
Unhappiness

Why Your Immune System Needs Boosting

Here are a few reasons for boosting your immune system:

1 Your immune system determines how fast you age.

2 Your immune system fights off the viruses, bacteria and other organisms which try to attack you and cause illness, from the common but irritating ones, like the cold, flu and thrush, to the more rare but often deadly ones like Legionnaire's disease and AIDS.

3 Your immune system has the power to destroy cancer cells as they are formed.

4 Your immune system empties your body's dustbin every day, getting rid of dead cells, dead invaders, and toxic chemicals.

5 Your immune system offers protection from radiation and chemical pollutants.

6 If you do not look after your immune system it could lose control and cause allergy problems or autoimmune diseases, like arthritis.

7 With a struggling immune system you are ill more often, more seriously, for more days of your life.

8 With a strong immune system you are almost invincible and should be able to lead a long, healthy and active life.

Essentially life is for living and giving, for learning and loving, for achieving and enjoying and no one wants to waste more time than they have to being sick.

2

HOW STRONG IS YOUR IMMUNE SYSTEM?

I t's your body, it's been with you since before you were born, yet how well do you know it? How well do you communicate with it? Just as we all have different fingerprints, so too do we all have different physical, nutritional and emotional requirements and different early warning signs that something is amiss. Your body will tell you if it is getting too many toxic minerals or not enough nutritional ones. It will tell you if it is under stress, not getting enough exercise or sleep. It will tell you if it is being invaded by viruses or bacteria, but do you understand what it is telling you? Do you recognise the symptoms early enough? Do you do anything about it?

It is important to get to know what the usual you is like and to be aware of any slight symptoms which are different for you. When an attack or insult is only slight, the symptoms will be mild. As the attack becomes more persistent or aggressive, so the strength of the symptoms will increase. How loud does your immune system have to shout before you take any notice? The earlier you recognise the symptoms the faster you can take corrective action and the more likely you are to avert the battle and avoid becoming ill. Use the list of early warning signs on the next page, pick out the ones that apply to you and add any others that you know of, or come across as you become aware of them. Get to know yourself. It's the longest lasting relationship that you can have.

Single symptoms show localised problems or changes which may or may not be significant, eg. a painful ear could mean an ear infection which if not treated could be serious, whereas if you are ravenously hungry after a long walk in this country, this is a perfectly normal request by the body for more fuel rather than a warning of a possible tapeworm inhabiting your gut! Combinations of symptoms are often more significant. Either way, pay attention to your body's messages and try to supply its needs.

Is Your Immune System Overloaded?

- Are you often ill with common infections?
- Do you often feel tired and lacking in energy?
- Do you find it difficult to concentrate and to be interested and enthusiastic about life?
- Are you unhappy with any major aspect of your life?
- Do you find difficulty mixing with other people?
- Do you feel either isolated or trapped?
- Do you easily get upset, angry, anxious, irritable etc.?
- Do you take very little exercise?
- Have you had any major changes in life recently?
- Do you take any drugs or medicines?
- Are you dependent on cigarettes, coffee or alcohol?
- Do you have allergy problems?
- Are you overweight?
- Are you overweight and can't seem to lose it no matter how much you count calories?
- Are you underweight but seem to be able to eat whatever you like but not get fat?
- Do you eat a lot of refined, convenience foods?
- Do you rarely eat raw fruit or vegetables?
- Do you eat a lot of processed, snack foods in between or instead of meals?
- Are you unsure of what supplements you need?
- Do you already have a medical condition that is pulling you down?
- Do you get a lot of vague aches and pains?
- Are you often tense, irritable and find it difficult to let go and relax?
- Do you sleep badly?

The more times you answered yes, the more strain there is on your immune system.

Early warning signs of an immune system in trouble

Do you notice any changes in the following ?

Hair	fall, texture, dry or greasy, colour, growth.
Head	dull ache, pain on movement, flushing or burning sensations, feelings of floating, fogginess, dizziness.
Eyes	yellowed whites, bloodshot, itchy, scratchy, dull not sparkling, pain on movement from side to side, watery, change in vision, tiredness.
Ears	itchy, painful, noises inside, sounds appearing far away whilst own voice is loud, flaking skin.
Nose	running, itching, sore, congested, difficulty breathing, loss of smell, sneezing.
Mouth	bad taste, bad breath, coated tongue, ulcers, loss of taste, bleeding gums, bad teeth, sore tongue, difficulty chewing, change in quantity of saliva.
Neck	stiffness or pain on movement.
Throat	sore, painful to swallow, swollen glands.
Digestive	indigestion, gas, burning sensations, bloatedness, pain, constipation, tract diarrhoea.
Muscles	weakened, painful, numb, tingling, flabby, tense, easily injured.
Joints	stiffness, weakness, tremors, swelling, pain.
Skin	spots, rashes, colour change, dry flaky, blotchy, new or altered moles or body hair, dull, tight, flabby, bloated, body odour.
Nails	ridged, brittle, white spots, blue tinged, split.
Energy levels	higher, lower, intermittent, erratic, hyperactive, dependent on food, coffee or stimulant intake.
Sleep	poor, broken, heavy, restless, excessive sweating, altered dreaming.
Mental	poor concentration, poor memory, lack of interest, forgetfulness.
Hunger	ravenously hungry, off food, food cravings.
Mood change	depressed, sad, up and down, irritable, frustrated, despairing, trapped.

How about your habits?

Habits can be boring. They are things that you do regularly, often without thinking about what you are doing. Unhealthy habits are easy to slip into and it can be interesting and fun to identify your unhealthy habits and change them for something new and healthier. Over two and a half thousand years ago, the Greek philosopher, Pythagoras and the Jewish prophet, Daniel, linked bad habits to disease and destruction.

Pythagoras is reputed to have said, "Man, by his habits, sets into motion those agencies which will eventually destroy him". This statement is timeless, so consider your habits. Which are destroying you? Which are helping you? What would you like to change? Consider the sample below.

Habits - Good and Bad. Which apply to you?

- Do you get angry quickly?
- **Do you avoid processed foods as much as possible?**
- Do you drink water from the hot tap?
- **Do you get natural light (not from behind glass) on you, especially your eyes, every day?**
- Do you eat a lot of fried foods?
- **Do you avoid artificial colours and flavours in food and drink?**
- Do you eat a lot of spicy, highly flavoured food?
- **Do you feel competent and confident?**
- Do you use the car, even for short trips?
- **Do you eat some fruit and vegetables every day?**
- Do you get irritated easily?
- **Do you enjoy life?**
- Do you eat cakes and biscuits every day?
- **Do you know which food supplements you need?**
- Do you add sugar to your food?
- **Are you satisfied with what you are doing with your life?**
- Do you eat a lot of convenience food?
- **Do you have a firm religious belief?**
- Do you get depressed easily?
- **Do you eat about 20% of your food raw?**
- Do you eat out in restaurants a lot?

- **Do you smile and laugh often?**
- Are you addicted to any food (especially tea, coffee, alcohol, sugar, wheat or chocolate)?
- **Do you make friends easily?**
- Do you cry or feel like crying often?
- **Do you have a satisfying sex life with only one partner?**
- Do you ever have time to eat properly?
- **Do you include a quiet period in your daily life (relaxing or meditating in silence)?**
- Do you find it difficult to make or keep friends?
- **Do you include oats two or three times in the weekly diet?**
- Do you find it difficult to express your feelings?
- **Do you sleep well?**
- Do you avoid fibre - containing foods?
- **Do you feel loved and in love?**
- Do you suffer with sunburn often (weather permitting)?
- **Do you take food supplements?**
- Do you feel lonely, trapped and unloved?
- **Do you pray or meditate?**
- Are you overweight?
- **Do you swim once a week or more?**
- Do you add salt to your food daily?
- **Do you eat fish once or twice a week?**
- Do you use a lot of household, cosmetic or garden chemicals?
- **Do you include exercise (other than swimming) in your daily routine?**
- Do you have a frustrating sex life?
- **Do you eat wholegrains other than wheat regularly?**
- Do you smoke?
- **Do you wash frequently, but without soap?**
- Do you use drugs?
- **Do you restrict meat to less than 2lb per person per week?**
- Do you have sex with more than one partner?
- **Are you happy with the shape of your body?**
- Do you drink more than one measure of alcohol a day?
- **Do you clean your teeth after every meal?**
- Do you use the pill or antidepressants?

- **Do you drink more than two pints of fluid a day (excluding alcoholic drinks)?**
- Do you use laxatives or antacids regularly?
- **Do you take some mono or polyunsaturated fat every day?**
- Do you use appetite suppressants, sleeping pills or pep pills?
- **Do you eat nuts and seeds weekly?**
- Do you dwell on the day's problems in bed at night?
- **Do you enjoy being with your family?**
- Do you live or work near electricity pylons, overhead power lines, or radio transmitters?
- **Do you keep animal fat to less than 15% of your total diet?**
- Is your daily life conducted in a noisy atmosphere?
- **Do you enjoy your work?**
- Do you live or work in a smoky atmosphere?

Obviously the odd lines are the unhealthy habits and the even ones the healthier habits.

How immune power improves your health

Health is defined by the World Health Organisation as a state of complete physical, mental, emotional and social well being not merely the absence of disease or infirmity.

By this ideal standard all of us are in various stages of 'unhealthiness' for much of our lives. Although we may never reach perfection of this ideal we are all capable of striving for excellence and can at least avoid a great deal of illness.

With an out of condition immune system you can expect to be ill more often and more seriously for more days of your life. There are always plenty of disease-causing bacteria, viruses, fungi and other organisms hanging around, either in the body or in the environment, just waiting for their chance to attack a nice juicy human. They are part of life in this world; we cannot avoid them but we do have a system for coping with them. We have several armies of immune cells which recognise these invaders, attack them and hopefully destroy them before they destroy us. If our personal immune system is overworked, inefficient or undernourished it will not be able to equip an army able to recognise the enemy and destroy it; that is when we develop disease. How long the disease affects us depends on how long it takes for the immune system to become effective and fight back.

By maintaining our immune system in peak condition, it is, at best, possible to avoid symptoms of illness completely and, at worst, it is possible to put together an effective fighting force quickly so that the illness is less severe and does not last as long.

The immune system can destroy cancer cells. We all make these cells but keep them under control. It is when the cancer cells are formed at a rate at which the immune system cannot cope that cancer becomes a problem.

Similarly, as long as the immune system is working correctly, there is no problem with autoimmune diseases. It is only when the immune system goes wrong and does not recognise self as self any more that autoimmune diseases occur and the army starts attacking the body's own cells as well as its enemies.

Part 2

UNDERSTANDING IMMUNITY

3

THE IMMUNE ARMY AND THE BATTLEGROUND

Basically, immunological battles can occur anywhere in the body, and can involve all organs and tissues, the blood system, etc. We do have a fixed defence framework within the body, called the lymphatic system, outlined in the diagram.

The lymphatic system

The *lymphatic system* is a network of vessels which branches throughout the body and contains a clear fluid called *lymph*. Unlike the blood system, there is no pump to force the lymph around. Movement of this fluid is instead brought about by muscle contraction; hence exercise is important in preventing a sluggish immune system.

Areas of special importance in the immune system are the thymus gland, the bone marrow, blood, spleen, liver (the Kupfer cells), the pituitary and adrenal glands, tonsils, adenoids, appendix, the intestinal Peyer's patches and the lymph nodes.

The *lymph nodes*, or lymph glands, lie on the lymphatic vessels and are areas of high immunological activity, favourite battle grounds when war is underway. As you can see from the diagram, the body is, for defence purposes, divided into six areas. Each area has its own nodes (where much of the fighting takes place); these nodes become the 'enlarged glands' which appear in many infections. Each area tries to confine such immunological battles to within its own boundaries; if, however, an individual's defence is weak, other areas become involved and infected. The pituitary gland in the brain co-ordinates all the immune activity in the head and the neck area, while the central core is the main defence headquarters.

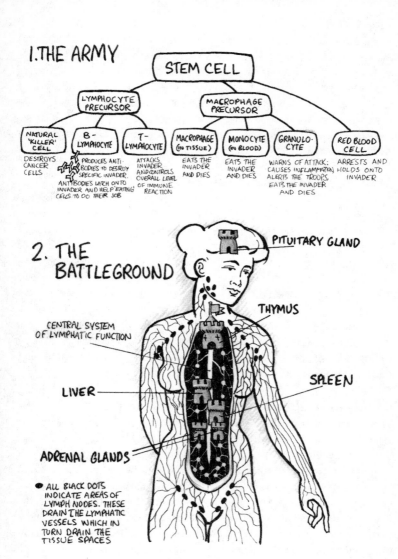

The Immune Army and Battleground

The thymus

The thymus is the master gland of the immune system, situated behind the breast bone in the chest. It is very active before and around the time of birth, but begins to decrease in size and activity from puberty onwards. *Growth hormone* stimulates it, while sex hormones depress it. It is essential for all T cell activity, and is responsible for distinguishing friend from foe. Thymus activity is closely linked to the rate at which we age. In old age the larger and more active the thymus, the more youthful and resistant we are to disease.

Macrophages and phagocytes

Throughout the entire lymphatic system there are cells which are fixed to their posts and not allowed to wander out of their allocated area. These cells are called *macrophages* and they are programmed to search and sift through whatever passes by them and literally to eat anything that is rubbish or foreign. This process is called *phagocytosis*, and *phagocytes* are any cells that feed in this way. This means, in effect, that the whole of our body has guards posted around it whose sole purpose is to look for, and get rid of, any unwanted material.

Macrophages and other phagocytic cells in the blood and lymph use this form of feeding to get rid of any of our dead or broken cells and any rubbish or invaders. They get breakfast, lunch, dinner, snacks and midnight feasts, whilst protecting us from attacks.

Blood and blood cells

The blood is an important part of the defence system. It is made up of a clear yellow fluid, called the plasma, and the blood cells which are suspended in the fluid.

Blood is pumped around the entire body by the heart. Major blood vessels branch into smaller ones and eventually into a network of capillaries so that blood can reach every tissue. It takes oxygen from the lungs to every tissue, and transports the waste carbon dioxide away. It carries food to every tissue and cleans up afterwards, by taking waste to the kidneys and liver for eventual removal. It also distributes heat to all parts of the body. Finally it provides us with a mobile fighting force of white blood cells which are our main immune soldiers. When in good working order, we are able to synthesise around 2,000 new immune cells every second. That's some fighting force, and would be quite a deterrent if germs had any brains.

The *white blood cells* or *leucocytes* are present in the lymph as well as in the blood. Some can even squeeze into tissue to fight an infection.

Platelets

Platelets or thrombocytes are small fragments in the blood that are important for our defence because they can get stuck together and coagulate the blood where there is an injury, so preventing all 5 litres pouring out of the hole and leaving the body empty! The plasma contains a substance called fibrin which forms a mesh at the site of the wound, to which the platelets stick. There are between 150,000 and 400,000 platelets per cubic millimetre of blood.

Red blood cells

The red blood cells or *erythrocytes* are the most common little robots in the blood. There are some 25 million million in the body of an adult man, or about 5 million per cubic millimetre. I call these cells robots rather than soldiers because, two or three days before they mature and leave the bone marrow where they are formed, they squeeze out their nuclei; this removes their ability to divide again and to form new cells, and they are therefore destined for destruction about four months later.

After leaving the bone marrow they enter the blood stream, where their role is really only to act as a receptacle for carrying oxygen around the body. They do however, have suction pads or docking points on their surface. Should any of the 25 million million of them come across anything alien whilst they are on their oxygen delivery rounds, they can use these to arrest it and deliver it to a more senior member of the immune army for sentencing and despatch.

White blood cells

There are 3 main types:
1 Granulocytes
  Granulocytes are further divided into:
* Polymorphonuclear neutrophils (PMN's for short)
* Eosinophils
* Basophils

The *eosinophils* and *basophils* make up at most 6% of the total white blood cell count and are significant in allergies and worm infections.

Polymorphonuclear neutrophils (polymorphs or PMN's) are very small cells with multilobed nuclei, and make up 50 to 70% of the total white cell count. They are phagocytic, gobbling up the foreign bacteria that they come across.

Inside the *polymorphs* there are little sealed bags called *lysosomes* which are broken when extermination is needed. Enzymes released from these bleach the alien to death, but are also strong enough to digest the little PMN's as well. Pus found at the site of an infection is a mixture of dead bacteria and the dead PMN army that fought so hard to conquer the enemy.

2 Monocytes and macrophages
Monocytes are much larger than red blood cells and polymorphs, they are essentially the same as macrophages.

Although less than 10% of the total white blood cell count consists of macrophages, they are very important. They destroy invaders by phagocytosis and clean our blood, tissues and lymph like efficient selective vacuum cleaners. They are also major chemical factories, capable of making at least 40 different enzymes and immune proteins needed as weapons for the destruction of enemies. The peacetime chemical activities include making enzymes necessary for clotting of the blood and fat transport.

They are not necessarily killed during an attack and they may live for some time, but even in death they are useful as they are broken down, cannibal - style, by other macrophages and used as food.

3 Lymphocytes
Lymphocytes make up somewhere between 20% and 30% of the total white cell count (depending on the degree of infection of the person at a given time). They are the most competent and versatile group for getting rid of unwanted guests. There are around one million lymphocytes in the average adult body and the principal centres for their production are the lymph nodes, spleen, thymus, Peyer's patches, appendix and other lymphoid tissue; 80% of these cells survive 100 to 200 days.

Lymphocytes have a memory system, so that when second or third invasion by the same kind of bug occur, the immune system can move into action right away, instead of wasting time relearning old lessons. Because a reinfection can be tackled immediately it is usually much milder than an initial attack. Lymphocytes have a special method of rapid cell division when under attack, so that they can produce reinforcements almost immediately and you hardly know that you have been into battle. This rapid division is very nutrient dependent; for example, vitamin C levels are crucial. All lymphocytes can move around between tissues, lymph or the blood stream; none remain fixed, and so a body-wide distribution and memory are ensured.

There are two major types of lymphocytes:
• **T Cells**
• **B Cells**

T lymphocytes

Not all *T lymphocytes* are the same. There are different jobs done by different groups, but all of the T cells have passed through the thymus (the master immune computer) for programming before they are let loose on the body. Some are unarmed and cruise around on surveillance duty, whilst others carry deadly warheads. They provide the initial response to viruses and tumour cells and the rejection of transplants. It takes three to four days after recognition for the T cells to get their act together and attack.

• *T helper cells* (known as TH or T4 cells) help other members of the immune army, but are not armed themselves. They are the body's safeguard against mistakes. If there is a possible invader of questionable identity, it is these T helper cells which determine their fate. These helper cells are also responsible for verifying an invasion and switching the immune system on. The human immunodeficiency virus that causes AIDS likes to invade these cells, so the victim ends up with few of these helper cells.

   This loss, (much simplified) tricks the body into leaving the immune system switched off, even though there is a major invasion taking place.

• *T suppressor cells* (also known as TS or T8 cells) switch off the immune system (both B and T cells) when an infection has passed and recovery is complete. Like the helper cells, the T suppressor cells are not armed.

• *Cytotoxic T cells* come complete with destructive powers. Their special duty is to search out viruses, etc., which have hidden themselves inside your cells. Most of the body's immune army, when they come across a healthy cell, recognise it and leave it alone, but the cytotoxic T cell has the ability to seek out and destroy any of the body cells that have a traitor within. They have very strong enzyme 'missiles' which break up and destroy the infected cell. Although they do have a specific target, there is bound to be some damage caused to surrounding cells by the use of such strong weapons.

• *Lymphokine - producing T cells* also have missiles, but these are aimed at invaders which move in between the body's own cells. Both these and the cytotoxic cells stimulate an increase in activity of the macrophages, as the lymphokines and other chemical weapons do cause a lot of destruction when they have to be used and there are a lot of dead cells and debris to be cleared away by the normal phagocytic method.

B lymphocytes

B lymphocytes deal mainly with bacteria and with reinfections by viruses that have been encountered before. Attack by a B cell is thus very specific; furthermore, it often requires help from other immune cells.

The task of a B cell is to take an invading bug into the tissues, and there to ascertain its exact size and shape. It then tailor-makes a straight jacket, called an antibody, that will fit that bug and no other. Finally it gets a factory-style production line going which manufactures thousands more of these antibodies which are released back into the body.

These, in turn, attach to the bacteria which triggered the reaction in the first place. They search out their targets and attach to them like mini guided missiles. The invader becomes harmless and is held until macrophages or PMN's come along to devour it.

Antibodies

Each *antibody* is a Y-shaped protein with a clamp or a straight jacket on each of the two top arms. Although they are made en masse in one of five basic patterns, the end product is tailored specifically to one bug only.

The pattern for these receptors is held in memory banks, so that they can be made to order immediately should reinfection occur. This, of course, is the principle upon which vaccination is based, where small quantities of a killed or altered bug are injected into the bloodstream so that antibodies can be made to it; on subsequent infection by the bug that causes the disease, the body can act right away and kill it before it has a chance to get hold and reproduce.

When first infected it can take five days for an antibody response. Peak levels of antibodies are then recorded around 14 days. However, on reinfection, antibodies can often be detected within 48 hours, and they persist much longer.

Antibodies are often referred to as *immunoglobulins*. Each molecule of immunoglobulin is made up of two identical light chains (around 2000 amino acids each) and two identical heavy chains (which are twice as long). Heavy chains are linked together by what are known as disulphide bonds. This is very significant as some chemicals alter or break disulphide bonds. Fluoride is a good example of such a chemical - immunoglobulins are very susceptible to this type of poison.

These immunoglobulins or antibodies are produced by the B lymphocytes in response to infection. The infecting agents or *antigens* are presented to the B lymphocytes by the T lymphocytes, and these B cells then mature and produce one of five antibody patterns: *IgG, IgA, IgM, IgD* and *IgE*.

IgG

This is the most abundant antibody, forming 75% of the total serum immunoglobulin level. PMN's and macrophages have receptor sites for the trail part of the IgG antibody and so can attach and eat the antibody and its captives when it is ready.

IgG is required by cells which are active in destroying cancer cells, although, unfortunately, they are also involved in transplant rejection and autoimmune diseases.

IgG is actively transported across the placenta and gives both the fetus and the new born baby (up to six months) protection. The infant usually starts making his own IgG at around three months, which is when immunisation programmes often begin.

IgA

This type of antibody is found in serum and mucus secretions of the respiratory, genito-urinary and intestinal tracts, where exposure to foreign substances is common. Being protein, immunoglobulins are liable to be digested by the gut enzymes, but IgA can produce a 'secretory piece' which gives it some protection against this. In gastric juices, 80% of the immunoglobulins are IgA. IgA is often low in those who suffer from respiratory and gastro - intestinal infections.

IgA's memory and specifity is poor in comparison with the other antibodies, but this is necessary, particularly in the gut, otherwise you could become irrevocably sensitised to almost anything you eat - a boiled egg, for example. People who suffer from food allergy problems probably have malfunctioning IgA; they become over sensitive to certain foods which, in any other person, would not be harmful. Hayfever sufferers are similar; pollen is not really harmful, but some people have a violent reaction to these usually harmless particles.

IgM

IgM is the largest and most primitive immunoglobulin. Its size makes it useful for picking up loads of small antigens, which it can manage ten at a time.

IgD

Not a lot is known about IgD, but levels are high in the disease of malnutrition, kwashiorkor.

IgE

IgE is attracted to mast cells (cells involved in allergic response) and basophils. It is associated with all forms of allergy including hayfever, asthma, hives, itching, rhinitis, etc. People who suffer from allergies usually make too much IgE, and allergic tendency can be passed on to children, although the allergy may not take on the same symptoms and form.

I. THE ARMY

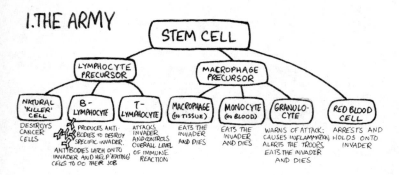

The Immune Army

A summary of the weapons of immunity

• Red blood cells merely arrest invaders and pass the package to the white blood cells to deal with.

There are several types of white blood cells:

• Macrophages and polymorphs eat the enemy.

• Eosinophils and basophils cause inflammation and warn of infection.

• B lymphocytes attack specific targets. They need one or two weeks to make a good supply of antibodies and to remember their targets so that they can supply antibodies faster should there be a second attack.

• T lymphocytes regulate the immune system and decide whether it goes into battle or withdraws. Some T lymphocytes attack.

Finally, lets look at three terms that often cause confusion:

• *Antigens* are anything which provokes an antibody response. Bugs which can cause disease are said to be antigenic because their presence in the body causes the B cells to make antibodies to help destroy them.

• *Antibiotics* are a sort of mercenary chemical force which is sometimes sent in by doctors to help combat a bacteria infection. Antibiotics are not made in the body, and should not be confused with antibodies - they are not the same thing at all.

4

HOW THE IMMUNE
SYSTEM WORKS

Immunity literally means being exempt from getting something. The immune system has to be able to destroy anything which threatens the body. When you are in good health, everything is in balance. Everything is working in harmony with everything else, resulting in a complete and healthy whole.

When we are sick, the balance is lost. The immune system battles conscientiously to restore the balance. If it succeeds, we are well again. If it does not, however, other influences may take advantage of the upset system and join the battle, so putting the system out of balance in other ways. As long as the immune system stays in control, the battle will eventually be won and order restored.

Infections

Bacteria, viruses, fungi, protozoa, parasites and worms are freely available in our world. There is no way of avoiding them completely while still living a normal life. The answer is to get the balance. Coming into contact with a disease - causing bacteria bug does not automatically give it the right to take over. We constantly live with the fungus that causes thrush, for example, or the bug that causes pneumonia. Most of us have a immune system that keeps these under control, as long as we don't alter the balance. Taking a lot of antibiotics that kill our friendly bacteria will allow the irritant fungus (not affected by the antibiotics) to grow into spaces where the friendly bugs would normally be. The result is thrush. If our immune system has been fighting a serious disease and we are recuperating, the pneumonia bug can seize its opportunity and attack whilst the body's defences are low, causing serious pneumonia.

Many diseases, including the common cold, are infections and we should try not to pass these on to others, in particular the very young, the sick and the elderly. It is a poor friend who has an infection and goes and visits someone in hospital who has just had a baby, or has undergone surgery. Keep your unfriendly bugs to yourself.

Adaptations for certain exceptions

It is no good destroying everything that is foreign that enters your body. We need food, for example, to live, but it is foreign, non - self; the gut therefore has to let its immune system adapt so that foreign food material can pass through unheeded. We can usually eat an egg with no ill effects, but the egg could not be injected straight into the blood stream - the immune system there would attack it immediately.

In order for us to reproduce, foreign sperm has to enter the female body. The sperm, that is non - self, therefore has to come complete with local immune suppressors so that it can survive. The pregnant woman's whole immune system has to change a lot in order to allow a completely different body to live inside her for nine months.

Many bacteria are unfriendly, but not all of them; some are necessary for our normal everyday existence, and it is very important that our immune system does not attack them. When our friendly gut bugs are destroyed with antibiotics, we are left open to attack by fungi and other pathogens (harmful organisms). We need our friendly neighbourhood bugs in the gut, on the skin, in the genitourinary tract and other mucous membranes so that the foreigners cannot establish themselves and change the environment to our disadvantage.

At a more fundamental level, civil war must be avoided - the immune system must not attack its own men (a difficult task when there are several million of them). It is also important that weapons intended for use on invaders do not accidentally destroy our own troops; they need to be carefully disarmed for day to day living.

There are two main types of immunity: nonspecific and specific.

Non - specific immunity

We will deal with the non specific or general immunity first.
• **Immunity due to species**
All living things are not susceptible to all disease causing organisms.

Have you ever seen a dog with a cold or the measles? Probably not, because the germs that cause these diseases do not affect the dog. The rabies virus, however, will attack both man and dog once it can get inside the skin, so this disease is transmissible through a bite or a wound.

• The rat is not susceptible to the diphtheria bacteria and can live quite happily in sewers, whilst guinea-pigs are highly susceptible to the disease and would not survive long in such a environment. The myxomatosis virus favours rabbit, whilst the bacteria causing leprosy and syphilis prefer man. We humans do not suffer from fowlpox or potato blight - we are naturally immune.

• Immunity due to genetics
There are some illnesses which are genetically determined. Most of us, for example, do not suffer from haemophilia. It is not an infection; you cannot catch it; you cannot make it go away by altering diet or exercise. It is genetically determined who has it and who does not.

• Biochemical barriers to infection
We have chemicals inside us which destroy unwanted bugs and other substances. Their effect is general, not specific to any one kind of bug.

• Lysozyme
Blood, eye fluids and many of our cells carry an enzyme called *lysozyme* which is just such a chemical. It is sometimes called the natural antibiotic, as it destroys bacteria. Fleming discovered both lysozyme and penicillin. Lysozyme is found in dilute solution in body fluids. In the immune cells, however, it is concentrated in special little packets called *lysozomes*. When these burst, this concentrated lysozyme is released and kills the invading bacteria. It will, of course, destroy some of the body cells as well, so it is important that these packets of concentrated lysozyme remain intact and only get broken in order to attack disease causing bacteria.

• Interferon
Interferon is an antiviral agent, but again it is non-specific, ie it will act against any virus that it finds lurking about. It prevents a virus from multiplying inside the cell, probably by closing down the power source of that cell, and it can also prevent neighbouring cells from being infected. Most tissue cells can secrete interferon when infected, as long as they have significant vitamin C and manganese. Sometimes cells become altered (eg cancer cells); these may lose their ability to produce interferon and so are relatively easily invaded by other viruses.

The ability to make interferon is coded in our genes, our inherited material. Indeed the human interferon gene can now be synthesised; it is a very large gene of over 500 units or nucleotides, but when it is inserted into the bacterium called E.coli, the bacterium will make large quantities of interferon. This could obviously be very useful in medicine, although it is not the whole of the answer to the elimination of harmful viruses.

• Complement

The *complement system* is also non-specific. It comprises a group of proteins which come together, when stimulated, to bring about the destruction of unwanted material. Complement also seems to instigate the inflammatory process.

One method of complement fixation is dependent on calcium, the other on magnesium, but either method of activation is a valuable help to other parts of the immune system. Tumour cells, for example, can often survive in the presence of antibodies alone, but the addition of complement causes their cell membranes to become fragile and patchy, leading to cell death. In particular, complement proteins have been shown to be able to neutralise the herpes simplex virus.

In order to prevent their uncontrolled attack the complement proteins are usually found separated in the blood. It is only when they come together in the correct order, stimulated by a threatening situation, that they cause destruction. It is rather like taking a gun apart and only putting it together when there is something to shoot; it prevents it going off by accident.

• Other chemicals

Blood, sweat, tears and tissue fluids have various biochemically active anti - bug substances, such as properdin, beta lysins, basic proteins (such as protamine and histone), basic peptides (such as leukins and phaocytins) and basic polyamines.

Finally, the acidity of their skin and stomach secretions is a barrier to infection, as are sufficient zinc levels in seminal and amniotic fluid. Bile salts and essential fatty acids in the intestines also deter pathogens.

Physical barriers to infection

We have physical barriers that protect us from attack. Primarily, the skin keeps us in and, to a degree, separates us from the rest of the world. Secretions from its glands contain antifungi and antibacterial substances to protect the outer layer from attack. We also have many friendly bacteria on the skin's surface that prevent invasion by less friendly ones. As long as our skin is intact, we are relatively safe from the bugs which surround; however, if the skin has wounds, there is a risk of infection.

Obviously, to enable us to breathe, eat, secrete and reproduce, we have to have entrances into our bodies. These, in turn, have special skin surfaces and secretions that protect them. The damp, mucus membranes of the nose and respiratory tract, for example, along with the hairs and cilia (microscopic hairs), trap many would be invaders. Some well known respiratory bugs, like the ones causing influenza, interfere with the sweeping action of the cilia, which is why they are so successful.

There are no cilia in the gut, but mucus and peristalsis (the constant pushing movement of the gut) prevent much bacterial growth; the churning action and acidity of the stomach also prevent infection. Infection occurs when the mucous membrane is damaged or when peristalsis slows down (as in copulation), but can also be caused by food poisoning.

Tissues and cell walls, as well as the blood brain barrier and placental barrier, all prevent free exchange of material and so, to a degree, protect us from some things that might harm us. Coughing, sneezing and crying also get rid of potential harmful substances.

• **Temperature**

Many of the bugs that cause us to be ill are very fussy about the central heating system. For example, the bacillus that causes TB in humans will not infect cold blooded animals. Hens do not usually contract anthrax, but if their temperature is lower they can be infected. Bugs which cause gonorrhoea are killed above 40°C; before antibiotics became available, raising body temperature was a common treatment for this condition.

Macrophages and other immune cells work better at a temperature above normal body temperature; this is why fever often accompanies infection. If we try to lower a temperature, (providing it is not life threatening) we could be putting our immune cells at a disadvantage - mild fever aids the immune response. Obviously a very high temperature, over which the body appears to have lost control, must be lowered or it could be dangerous in itself.

• **Specific immunity**

Specific immunity is where the immune system acts against a particular bug or condition. It is usually divided into active and passive immunity and both are further divided into natural and artificial immunity.

• **Passive immunity**
Antibody cells or antitoxins can be transferred from an immune person to a non-immune person. This happens naturally when immunity is passed from mother to child via the placenta or in colostrum (a baby receives colostrum whilst breast feeding). Artificially, it may be used in medicine to treat tetanus, snake bite or those with immune deficient diseases. All passive immunity is short lived. Once the substance passed on to the non-immune person is used up, the beneficial effects are lost.

• **Active immunity**
This is where the body's own immune cells recognise a specific bug or substance and react to it. It has a memory, to recognise and deal with the problem on subsequent occasions. So B and T cell activity, as well as some macrophage activity, is specific. Natural active immunity occurs during infection, and artificial active immunity happens when we are immunised.

Nutritional support

Natural antibiotic production, production of complement proteins, ability to carry out phagocytosis and to digest the prey are dependent on vitamin C, so it is easy to see that an increased consumption of this vitamin at the time of infection (rather than at the time of symptoms) is crucial. The vitamin C at the time of infection immediately increases the protection: taken a day or so later, it will be far less effective.

Complement production is calcium and magnesium dependent, whilst interferon production is manganese dependent. Calcium is also needed for fever production which aids our immune soldiers. All three nutrients are commonly deficient in the refined diet, although we are getting much more conscious about calcium these days.

We have seven main ways of defending ourselves. As we have just seen, methods two, three and four are all impaired by something as simple as vitamin C deficiency. The effect of nutrition on the immune system and how we can support it will be dealt with in a later chapter.

5

UNDERSTANDING AUTOIMMUNITY

Autoimmunity is when the body's own immune system attacks itself, rather like a civil war, where an army attacks its own men. Possibly it no longer recognises its own men. To understand this we need to be familiar with the theory of how the immune system recognises an invader and recognises self.

Distinguishing friend from foe

How do the defending white cells know what to attack and what to protect? The answer lies in the master computer, the thymus. Since before you were born it has been giving all your cells an 'identity disc' and a code which is recorded in its 'memory banks'. A language analogy helps the understanding of what goes on here.

Think of your body as a country where every individual cell has been taught to speak the same language - English. We can immediately recognise someone from another country if they speak a different language. When your immune army recognises a foreigner, it immediately assumes that it is there to attack and so arrests the invader and destroys it.

There are three problems here:

1 The foreigner may not be hostile, it may even be trying to be helpful, eg a new heart transplanted. The intention is good, the old heart is faulty, or even packed up altogether, but in order to put in one which will not be recognised as self, doctors have to give immune suppressing drugs or the foreign heart is rejected.

2 A French person could come into this country and speak perfect English and we may not recognise them as foreign. A similar sort of situation occurs if a virus gets into your body and manages to get inside one of your cells before it gets caught. The immune army recognises your

cell, but not necessarily the invader within and so doesn't attack. Meanwhile, the virus takes over your cell's DNA and gets it to make its own instead so that your cell makes hundreds of new aliens! One of our cells, the cytotoxic T cell, is programmed to recognise this trick. When it picks up 'two languages' it destroys the virus and the host cell, so it's down to luck or an efficient immune system as to whether the virus gets discovered in time or not.

3 The third loophole is the American who just happens to have English as his native language as well. All of the immune cells recognise this cell as self and leave it alone. The bug which causes syphilis is like this. The antigen or identity disc on its surface is the same as that on some of your heart muscle cells, cardiolipin. Treponema, the bug which causes the damage, can create havoc in the body without being checked for some time. When the immune system eventually realises which traitor is doing the damage it attacks it, but in so doing also attacks the heart muscle which has the same code. It is now possible to destroy Treponema but it is important to do so before the body has recognised it as foreign, or else the immune system carries on attacking heart muscle even after the bug has been destroyed.

How does it write the identity disc?

Our cells obviously neither speak nor write, but they use amino acids instead of letters and therefore carry amino acid identity discs. A cell which carries a 'toes' or 'ship' or 'star' disc would be recognised as a skin, liver or whatever cell belonging to self and left alone by the immune army. Cells carrying 'posl', 'foyq' or 'qdbg' would be destroyed. It is a very clever system, but like all systems there are some problems:

1 A simple spelling mistake. If the body makes a mistake and writes 'stau' instead of 'star' then the immune cell will destroy it. This would be alright if it was an isolated error but if the body kept writing stau then an auto immune disease could follow, where our own immune cells destroy our own body cells because the label is wrong.

2 When the immune cells are overworked or understaffed, they may make a mistake and not recognise an 'English' word as English and so attack anyway, again attacking your own cells, so causing an autoimmune response.

Autoimmunity is, in effect, a language problem, misunderstandings due to errors in communication. It is surprising really that there aren't more errors. An average English speaking person has around 100,000 words available to him/her and we're always making communication mistakes! The immune system can synthesise around 10 million, and in theory, antibodies can be made to all of them, although not everyone can. There are often large gaps in vocabulary.

Examples of autoimmune conditions are, pernicious and haemolytic anaemias, Addison's disease, systemic lupus erythematosis and rheumatoid arthritis. Ulcerative colitis is possibly caused by confusion between a marker on the colon (large intestine) and a bacterial inhabitant of the gut, E. coli. The immune cells attack both causing inflammation of the colon. Another interesting example is the sperm, the hidden antigen. Because there is no sperm present at birth, it is not marked as self and so are kept separate from the immune cells. In a rare complication of mumps, it is possible that the virus attacks the separating membrane, the immune cells fail to recognise the sperm as self and attack. Protein from the lens of the eye is similarly not recognised as self and so is protected from immune cells.

All of your cells have their own identity, function and needs. To stay healthy, all these individuals have to live together in harmony. Unfortunately there are many enemies which can upset this ideal state, from a poor diet and lack of exercise to environmental pollution, stress and overwork. When things get out of control errors or civil war can happen, so look after your inner army. One day your life and health may depend on it.

6

THE CAUSES AND CONSEQUENCES OF INFECTION

There is an underlying purpose for everything, including sickness. The usual purpose of physical or mental pain, is to draw attention to conditions of disharmony in the body, which require correction. Sickness, in body language, is telling us something is wrong. This could be an attack from external forces, like germs, or that we are doing something wrong which is causing us to malfunction.

When we are ill, our energy level drops because we are using energy to make more heat (our temperature goes up to improve activity of immune cells) and to instigate an immune response. Limbs ache or feel heavy because our available calcium and magnesium go to aid defence, so leaving our joints short of these essential minerals. There is usually loss of appetite and digestive problems as energy is needed for digestion and we don't have any spare. There is weight loss, because we use body stores for energy in the initial stages, not that from recently digested food, which is often not digested properly at this time anyway. The tongue becomes coated and the skin condition deteriorates, because these are major sites for removal of toxins.

There are several types of 'germ' waiting in the air, on food, in the water or just somewhere out there, needing a susceptible human to attack. Successful bugs will live in or on us for a while, replicate or reproduce and move on to humans new. Ironically, it's the less successful ones that kill their host, but that's not much consolation if those are the ones you've got!

Bacteria are the most well known causative agents of infectious diseases. Some try to evade the immune system by forming a protective capsule around themselves eg. the streptococci which cause sore throats and the bacteria that cause flu, pneumonia and meningitis. (There are viruses that can cause these illnesses too.) It works - they are very successful bacteria. Other bacteria have cell walls which are resistant to digestion by enzymes in our gut. Examples include Salmonella and the bacteria which cause TB (Mycobacterium tuberculosis) and leprosy (Mycobacterium leprae).

Other bacteria produce toxins, chemicals that attempt to immobilise the immune army, these include tetanus (Clostridium tetani), diphtheria (Corynebacterium diphtheriae) and cholera (Vibrio cholerae). The toxins produced by these and other bacteria persist and continue to do damage even after the bug has been killed. Some very successful bacteria like Pseudomonas, Listeria and E. coli only cause problems when the immune system is insufficient for some reason eg. immaturity, pregnancy, illness and old age. Not all bacteria have special talents and many can be dealt with very effectively by a competent immune system.

Viruses are the other common causative agents of infectious diseases. They are very small and have no magic bullet like the antibiotic to destroy them yet, so it's all down to the immune system. Our first line of defence against the virus is interferon. It is in an inactive form in the body most of the time because its action is not specific, ie. when it is activated by the presence of viral particles it makes a protein which, in effect, puts a stop on the copying of genetic material. This means that the virus cannot replicate and so is ineffective. It also stops the host cell from reproducing too, so the cell eventually dies. It's very potent stuff, but dependent on sufficient vitamin C and manganese.

Whilst the viruses that cause mumps, measles, smallpox, herpes, polio, typhus, yellow fever, etc. are in the blood, our antibodies can attack them. The success of the virus depends on its ability to get inside the host cell, where it can use the host's DNA to replicate itself. They play, in effect, one of the oldest tricks in the book - the Trojan horse. The only immune cell capable of recognising and destroying them once they have got this far is the cytotoxic T cell.

Some viruses stay in the body even after obvious infection has passed and can be reactivated at a later date causing the same or sometimes different symptoms. The herpes group of viruses, which cause cold sores, are a good example of this. Chicken pox virus can present itself again as shingles at a later date and usually after a low period, health wise.

Rhinoviruses (causing colds and flu) are very successful because they are constantly changing that recognition code on their surface, so as fast as medical science finds a cure for one type of flu, the bug changes and they have to start all over again on the new form.

Less than 20 protozoa cause disease in man and they aren't much of a problem in this country, although they are to the immune system and medical science because they have the same sort of cells that we have and so something that will attack them is liable to attack and destroy our own cells too. The most formidable ones are the insect borne protozoa which cause malaria (Plasmodium), sandfly fever (Leishmania) and sleeping sickness (Trypanosomes).

Toxocariasis is the main worm infection that is cause for concern in this country. It is passed to humans via the cat or dog. (Worms need a host other than man to reproduce in.) Pets should be wormed regularly because the Toxicara larvae burrow into blood vessels in the intestine, then go to the liver. Sometimes they can get into the lungs, eye or brain where they can cause irrevocable damage even though they usually die.

Athletes foot, ringworm and thrush are probably the most common fungal infections. Candida (fungus that causes thrush) in particular, is increasing rapidly, possibly due to antibiotic use, because when antibiotics are administered they kill all of the good bacteria in the body as well as the baddies but don't have any effect on fungi so they can reproduce and take up all of the living space that used to be inhabited by good bacteria, unless you are very quick to do something about it. After a course of antibiotics you should eat a lot of live yoghurt and take a B complex supplement in order to restore your body's good bacteria quickly and avoid the fungi moving in.

Persistent fungal infections, unchecked, cause the production of antibody complexes, which can lead to a build up of granulomas, which eventually calcify and could cause rheumatic-type pains in the joints.

Progress in combating infectious diseases

Robert Hooke and Antony van Leeuwenhoek opened the doors to the hidden world of microbes back in the eighteenth century, but their 'little new animals' were little more than acknowledged and observed, using very simple microscopes consisting of not much more than a biconvex lens. Leeuwenhoek's bacteria were thought to be the smallest living creatures until Martinus Beijerinck described 'a contagious living liquid' that caused tobacco mosaic disease in plants. It was not until the mid twentieth century that this was found to contain viral particles, tobacco mosaic virus.

Medical progress in combating infectious diseases has been outstanding since those first steps and the dawn of microbiology. Various epidemics used to wipe out whole populations. During the Justinian era, plague killed two thirds of the inhabitants of the major Roman cities. In Europe, leprosy was a much feared killer of the fourteenth century, as was the plague, then known as the Black Death, which wiped out twenty five million people in medieval Europe. It continued into the fifteenth century. The major sixteenth century killer was syphilis. Smallpox headed the death charts in the seventeenth and eighteenth centuries, whilst scarlet fever, measles and TB were the fears of the nineteenth. We now have the ability to prevent, treat or cure all of these. Possibly AIDS may go down in history as the disease of the twentieth century, although cancer and heart disease, (not infectious), take more lives.

The battle against infectious diseases was fought in stages. Robert Koch in the late nineteenth century came up with the 'germ theory' as a cause for these diseases. Joseph Lister in the early twentieth century discovered the antiseptics, (which saved many lives previously claimed by infections). It's a wonder any of us are still here! This discovery brought improvements in hygiene, living standards and public health.

Paul Erlich established the early basis for chemotherapy and became well known in his time for his 'magic bullets'. Alexander Flemming discovered penicillin which heralded the modern antibiotics. Edward Jenner introduced vaccination which provides resistance to specific diseases and is now widely used as a preventative measure.

In spite of these great leaps forward the bugs are fighting back and changing so that they are becoming resistant to our weapons. The search is on for alternative forms of treatment and prevention to combat these new or altered diseases. There are many routes to try, the obvious ones being finding something to kill or render harmless the causative agents, or ways of stimulating the body's own humoral and cellular defence mechanisms. Research is not only looking to the future, but it is also delving into the past and looking at methods which the ancient Greeks, Egyptians, Romans and existing primitive peoples used or use to kill or cure. The next section follows some of the natural lines of inquiry.

7

FIGHTING INFECTIONS NATURALLY

Prevention is better than cure and as Louis Pasteur said on his deathbed, "the host is more important than the invader". Increasingly we are becoming aware that we are more likely to succumb to bugs when already run down. So the best line of defence is to keep the immune system strong and provide it with what it needs when the next invader comes along. Everyone is exposed to germs that cause infectious diseases, but those with strong immune systems fight back more effectively and either avoid symptoms of the illness entirely or have a milder attack.

He who hesitates is lost. If you know you have just spent the morning talking to someone who has the flu, or the person next to you in the elevator sneezed and very kindly sent an army of cold bugs in your direction, get in there with the immune boosting nutrients and start the war yourself, rather than waiting until the next morning when you might wake up with a headache, sore throat, bloodshot eyes, itchy nose and feeling like the person you met yesterday.

If, however, you've missed your opportunity and the little bugs have settled in, made themselves comfortable, had a meal at your expense and are stealing your energy, turn up the heat and send in everything you've got to get them out. One day taking it easy in a conducive environment could make all the difference to the severity and duration of the illness, though I must admit that it would be very difficult to ring work with the rather feeble excuse of, "I won't be in today because I'm going to be ill due to this person that I met yesterday. I'll be in tomorrow as long as I get better, but if I come in today, I'll definitely be ill tomorrow and won't be in for the rest of the week".

However, back to turning the heat up. Immune cells work better at a higher temperature, this is why the body 'gets a temperature' when you are ill. When you have recovered, your temperature goes back to normal and the immune cells slow down again, on surveillance duty only. Keep your room warm, (remember the rest of your family may not want the central heating on full in August) and get some sleep. Sleep is the time when you heal and repair as well as produce chemicals which stimulate the immune system. Eliminate other energy robbers such as alcohol, smoke, strong light, loud sounds, overeating, highly processed foods, stress, sex and overexertion. Listen to your body, it may not want to eat for a day, but if the illness goes on for longer, there are some vital nutrients needed to replenish the troops.

Drink lots of water to dilute and eliminate toxins produced during the battle and to prevent dehydration. Avoid salt, mucus forming and fatty foods. Also avoid concentrated protein foods if you have any sort of stomach upset. A sensitive, damaged stomach could well develop food allergies at this time.

The A to Z of natural infection fighters

Vitamin A is one of the key immune-boosting nutrients. It helps to strengthen the skin, inside and out, and therefore acts as a first line of defence, keeping the lungs, digestive tract and skin intact. By strengthening cell walls it keep viruses out. Vitamin A has potential toxicity in large doses so levels above 10,000ius are recommended only on a short-term basis.

Aloe vera has immune-boosting, anti-viral and antiseptic properties, probably due to its high concentration of mucopolysaccharides. It's a good all-round tonic, as well as a booster during any infection.

Antioxidants are substances that detoxify 'free radicals'. These include vitamins A,C,E, beta-carotene, zinc, selenium and many other non-essential substances from silymarin (milk thistle), pycnogenol, lipoic acid, bioflavonoids and bilberry extract.

Artemesia is a natural anti-fungal, anti-parasitical and anti-bacterial agent, often used alongside caprylic acid for the treatment of candidiasis or thrush.

Astragulus is a Chinese herb renowned for all-round boosting immunity, high in beneficial mucopolysaccharides.

Beta-carotene is the vegetable source of pre-vitamin A and an antioxidant in its own right. It also has the advantage of being non-toxic,

Anti-Viral, Anti-Bacterial or Anti-fungal?
This chart tells you which

NUTRIENTS	ANTI-OXIDANTS	IMMUNE BOOSTERS	ANTI-VIRAL	ANTI-BACTERIAL
Vitamin A	✔	✔	✔	
Beta Carotene	✔	✔	✔	
Vitamin C	✔	✔	✔	✔
Vitamin E	✔	✔		
Selenium	✔	✔		
Zinc	✔	✔	✔	
Iron	✔	✔		
Manganese	✔			
Copper	✔			
B Vitamins	✔	✔		
L Cysteine	✔			
N A Cysteine	✔			
Glutathione	✔			
Lysine			✔	
Aloe Vera		✔	✔	✔
Astragalus	✔	✔		
'Power' mushrooms		✔	✔	
Echinacea		✔	✔	
St J's Wort		✔		✔
Garlic	✔	✔	✔	✔
Grapefruitseed			✔	✔
Silver			✔	✔
Tea Tree				✔
Artemesia				✔
Bee Pollen				✔
Cats Claw	✔	✔	✔	
Goldenseal				✔

Immune-boosting nutrients are good all year round, and especially if you're run down or exposed to people with infections. During an infection both the invader and our own immune army produce 'free radicals' to destroy each other. We can mine-sweep these dangerous chemicals with antioxidant nutrients. These are good for everybody at all times. Anti-viral, anti-bacterial and anti-fungal agents are best increased when dealing with a specific invader.

although it is prone to oxygen damage and is often unstable in supplements. Red, orange, yellow foods and fresh vegetables are the best sources. Carrot or watermelon juice is a great way to drink this all-round infection fighter.

Bee pollen is a natural antibiotic. It's probably best as a general tonic. Quality varies considerably as does contamination with lead. Unfortunately, bees are polluted too. So pick your source carefully and watch out for very cheap supplies. You may get what you pay for. Be careful if you're pollen sensitive or allergic to bee stings.

Vitamin C is an incredible anti-viral agent. In fact, no virus yet researched in vitro has survived the onslaught of high dose vitamin C treatment, from the common cold to HIV. In the test-tube even the HIV virus is eradicated within 4 days in a vitamin C rich environment. In a review of research studies using 1 to 6 grams of vitamin C daily, Drs Hemila and Herman found consistent evidence of shorter colds with less symptoms. During a viral infection the trick is to 'saturate' the bloodstream. Viruses cannot survive in such a vitamin C rich environment. Vitamin C is non-toxic. Too much can cause loose bowels. If this happens decrease the dose to your maximum bowel tolerance level.

Caprylic acid from coconuts is a specific anti-fungal agent, primarily used for eliminating the 'Candida albicans' organism responsible for thrush. You have to be a bit careful with the dose because as candida dies it produces toxins, so if you eliminate this problem too rapidly you can get worse before you get better. Anti-candida programmes are best done under the supervision of a qualified nutrition consultant.

Cats Claw, officially called Uncaria tomentosa, is a powerful anti-viral, antioxidant and immune boosting agent from the Peruvian rainforest plant,. It contains alkaloids, one of which is isopteridin, which has been proven to boost immune function. It is available as a tea or in supplements. As a tea it tastes good with added blackcurrant and apple concentrate.

Vitamin E is the most important fat-soluble antioxidant. It protects essential fats in nuts and seeds from going rancid. While you'll find it in nuts, seeds, wheatgerm and their cold-pressed oil, make sure they are fresh. Vitamin E is best supplemented every day with extra during an infection.

Echinacea is a great 'all-rounder' with anti-viral and anti-bacterial properties. It's the original Red Indian 'snakeroot'. The active ingredients are thought to be specific mucopolysaccharides.

Garlic contains allicin which is ant-viral, anti-fungal and anti-bacterial. It also acts as an antioxidant, being rich in sulphur-containing amino acids. There's no doubt it's an important ally in fighting infections, and a wise inclusion in one's diet as garlic eaters have the lowest incidence of cancer. Consider a clove or capsule equivalent for an easy guide to your daily dose.

Ginger is particularly good for sore throat and stomach upsets. Put six slices of fresh ginger in a thermos with a stick of cinnamon. Five minutes later you have a delicious and throat-soothing ginger and cinnamon tea. You can add a little lemon and honey for taste.

Glutathione & Cysteine are both powerful antioxidant amino acids. You'll find them in many all-round antioxidant supplements. During a prolonged viral infection they get depleted and may be worthy of extra supplementation. The most usable forms are reduced glutathione or N-Acetyl-Cysteine.

Grapefruit Seed Extract, also called Citricidal, is a powerful antibiotic, anti-fungal and anti-viral agent. The great advantage, however, is that it doesn't have much effect on the beneficial gut bacteria. It comes in drops and can be swallowed, gargled with or used as nose drops or ear drops, depending on the site of infection.

Lysine is an amino acid that helps get rid of the herpes virus. During an infection it's best to limit arginine-rich foods such as beans, lentils, nuts and chocolate.

Mushrooms such as shiitake, maiitake, reishi or ganoderma, traditionally believed by Chinese Taoist to confer 'immortality', have all been shown to contain immune-boosting polysaccharides. You'll find them added to some immune-boosting supplements and tonics, or you buy shiitake fresh in the supermarket or dried in health food stores.

Probiotics, as opposed to antibiotics, are beneficial bacteria that promote health. They are best used to restore balance in the digestive tract, for example, during a stomach bug. It's best to supplement extra during an bacterial infection. Specific strains found in the human digestive tract, called 'human strain bacteria', are now available. Watch out for ABCDophilus, a combination of three strains beneficial for infants and children. These have been shown to halve the recovery time from a bout of diarrheoa. Lactobacillus salivarius is a good strain for adults.

Selenium is an immune enhancing mineral that also acts as an antioxidant. It's rich in any food beginning with 'SE' including seafood and seeds, especially sesame. You'll find it included in most antioxidant supplements.

St John's Wort (hypericum) is particularly good for anything that penetrates the skin, such as a wound or skin infection. It's a good general tonic for the immune system.

Tea Tree Oil is an Australian remedy with antiseptic properties. Great for rubbing on the chest, in the bath, or steam inhaling and also helps keep mosquitoes away.

Zinc is the most important immune-boosting mineral, well worth upping during any infection. There's no question it helps fight infections. Zinc lozenges are also available for sore throats.

8

UNDERSTANDING
ALLERGIES

Allergy occurs when the body alters its normal immune response in some way, due to the presence of an allergen. Allergens are substances which bring about this immune response, and the odd thing about them is that they are not normally harmful; it appears to be the allergic individual who produces the wrong response. Ironically, many allergy sufferers are immune deficient in other ways as well.

In the case of contact sensitivities, such as allergy to nickel, jewellery or detergents, it is the lymphocytes and macrophages which over-react, but in most other allergies it is the antibody response which is over-reactive. The role of antibodies in allergy was not really well known until 1967, when the antibody IgE was discovered and associated with hayfever. IgE is not produced all over the body; it is made mainly in nasal and throat areas and the gut. It is believed that cross-links between IgE molecules and the surface of our mast cells (mast cells are specialised immune cells dotted around our tissues, packed with immunologically active chemicals) and basophils, cause the release of histamines, and it is the histamines, normally safely packaged inside the cells, which cause the soreness and itching and hence the need for anti-histamine medication. Vitamin C is a natural anti-histamine and can often be used to alleviate symptoms if the dose is right. IgA and IgG are also involved in allergic reactions.

Response to an allergen may be immediate or delayed, and is by definition an inappropriate or over-reaction of the immune system to inhaled or non-inhaled allergens. However, although a true allergy has to evoke an immune response, the term allergy is often broadened to include food intolerances.

Common Allergens

Inhalant	Dust, animal furs, moulds, perfumes; pollen, agricultural chemicals, gas, smoke, exhaust fumes, air conditioner or propellant gases.
Contact	Nickel, jewellery, soaps and detergents, bleaches, other household or industrial chemicals, cosmetics, animals, paints and dyes, glues.
Non-inhalant	Bites and stings from insects; drugs, e.g. penicillin, aspirin; foods especially fish, nuts, wheat, milk products, meat and eggs; artificial foods, especially colourings and flavourings.

Who suffers from allergies?

Whether due to an overall decline in our immune competence or to an increase in the burden on our immune system, or perhaps a bit of both, the cases of allergies are rapidly increasing.

Allergies can sometimes run in families. It is known that high total IgE levels can be inherited, as can faulty T cell response. The allergy, however, may not be the same down the generations. A child with asthmatic parents may be more prone to allergy, but she may suffer with eczema or hayfever instead.

Allergic symptoms also change with age. A baby with eczema may grow out of it only to become an adult who suffers from hayfever. Children often appear to suffer more from allergies than adults, but this may not actually be true; it could merely be that we are more aware of a child's symptoms and they have less control over them. An adult has learned how to cope with his recurrent migraine, but a child will perhaps be sick, and frightened of how she is feeling.

Common allergic reactions

These are usually grouped on the basis of the areas they affect.

The skin

Contact with an allergen can bring about various forms of dermatitis.

Hives

Hives are large whitish raised areas on the skin, with an itching red centre. They are often caused by a reaction to an insect bite, but they may be due to some other allergen. They sometimes come and go, in which case it is difficult to find the cause. The itching may be worse with exercise or any form of overheating including hot baths, tight clothes and emotional upset.

Eczema

This can be very itchy, and is usually worse in winter. It often starts as rough red patches on babies' cheeks; it may then disappear completely or come and go, spreading to other areas.

Wool can sometimes cause this or other types of skin reaction, but if the eczema persists there is nothing for it but to go through the whole list of possible allergens. It is helpful if you think back to the day before each incident occurred, particularly the first one.

It is far better to trace the cause of the eczema and remove it if possible, rather than resort to cortisone creams or other antihistamines (which are all immunosuppressants), but this is not always practical. Bubble baths and soaps are also best avoided, except for washing the hands and nails. Laundry soap has to be a suspect, and it may be necessary to use pure soap suds only for washing and then to put the washing through the machine again with no soap at all - just water. Exposure to some viruses, especially the cold sore virus, herpes, can make eczema worse. Even a smallpox or similar vaccination could be a real problem. Food is often a cause of eczema, and food allergies are worth investigating (see the next chapter).

Eczema is especially bad for children, as they automatically scratch the itch, which makes it even worse and can cause infection. Keep the fingernails short and clean, and perhaps buy cotton gloves to prevent involuntary scratching at night.

The head

Allergic symptoms may affect the eyes, nose, ears, lips or brain.

Migraine

Some forms of migraine can be caused by allergy, but it is not easy to find the cause; there are different triggers for different people and no one solution that works for everyone. It seems that allergens may cause the blood platelets to slow down the blood flow to the head by clumping together. A migraine attack follows, often causing a one-sided headache with feelings of nausea. Some people suffer so badly that they are forced to lie in a darkened room and hope for sleep. Attacks may last for hours or even days.

There are whole lists of foods and chemicals which have even cited as potential triggers for migraine, the most common being cheese, chocolate, yeasts, food flavourings and colourings, red wine, coffee, tea and sugar. Some medicines, like the pill, and some household chemicals have also been implicated.

Headaches may also be brought about by constriction of the blood vessels in the neck region due to some misalignment of the vertebrae; if so, an osteopath may be required to correct the problems. Involuntary constriction of the blood vessels is another cause and can be prevented by ensuring sufficient magnesium and niacin in the diet. Platelets may aggregate, leading to headaches, but they can be kept separated by having enough vitamins E, C, B6 and the essential fatty acids. Ensuring nutrient sufficiency and avoiding chemical triggers could avert many migraines. It all depends on the cause of the problem in the first place and, unfortunately, it often takes a lot of time and detective work to uncover the cause.

Hayfever

Hayfever causes a running nose, sneezing and watery eyes. Sufferers often have to clear their throat and breathe through the mouth; they may lose their sense of taste and smell to some degree. Hayfever can also cause altered moods, making people irritable, touchy, fussy, moody and listless; emotions can be involved, and children, in particular, cry very easily.

If you are a sufferer, things other than the pollen to which you are sensitive may bring on an attack, even pets. There is one school of thought that links susceptibility to hayfever with high wheat and sugar consumption; both of these are in the same family as the pollen which is known to trigger hayfever in this country. Many sufferers, although by no means all, relieve symptoms by switching to an unrefined diet low in wheat and sugar products.

Hayfever can also cause swelling inside the nose, the membranes becoming stretched and less resistant to infection; infection of ears, nose and throat is thus often an additional problem. The swelling and pressure in the nasal tissue can impair blood circulation, so dark circles as well as puffiness under the eyes are common features. The weakened nasal tissue is also likely to break and bleed, causing nose bleeds. Polyps may develop, especially if the hayfever sufferer is also sensitive to aspirin and foods containing salicylates - many herbs, spices and alcoholic drinks are high in salicylates, as are tea, coffee, cola and yeast foods.

Asthma

Aspirin and beta-blocker (blood-pressure-lowing drugs) sensitivity is more common in asthmatics than other people. Asthmatics are also more sensitive to metabisulphite (the preservative in wine and squashes) and tartrazine, as well as to polyunsaturated fats.

Hayfever can go on to develop into bronchial asthma, slipping, so to speak, from the nose to the chest. Asthma is not always due to allergy, but if the patient has previously suffered with eczema or hayfever, it probably is an allergic reaction. Most allergies are more common in females, but asthma is the exception, being two or three times more common in males.

Swelling occurs in the lining of the air tubes in the lung and the muscle around the air tube contracts, possibly due to an imbalance of calcium and magnesium in the diet; an asthmatic thus needs more dietary magnesium. With the swelling inside and squeezing outside, the air space in the tubes is much smaller and there is difficulty pushing the air out - hence the typical wheezing of asthma.

Wheezing causes a build-up of mucus in the lung. It is vital for an asthmatic to drink a lot, as this helps to keep the fluid thin; if it is allowed to become thick and rubbery, the problems get worse and may bring about vomiting, which in turn causes dehydration, so even more fluid is needed. It is important, however, not to drink things that will make this condition worse - ice-cold fluids, colas and coloured drinks can often cause problems.

Allergic symptoms may also affect other areas of the body, such as the hands, stomach, feet, blood vessels and bladder.

As with most allergic problems, it is a question of trying to find the triggers that bring about the condition. To complicate matters, there are often several triggers, not just one, which makes them not only difficult to find but also difficult to eliminate from the diet or immediate environment.

Other Conditions Associated with Allergy

Behaviour problems

Hyperactivity, vandalism and crime is going up all over the world and not just in proportion to the increase in population. Quite a few studies now show a link between diet and such antisocial behaviour (and it appears that unreal fears and phobias may also be associated with food or chemical sensitivity). Work has been done with prisoners and juvenile offenders which has shown that dietary modifications reduce aggressive and destructive behaviour. The link between allergies, nutritional imbalances and crime is only slowly being accepted in this country, but why are we so reluctant to accept what could be a very simple way to keep the crime rate down? We readily accept that alcohol and drugs destroy the body's reason and control, so why not chemicals in or sprayed onto foods? Animals put on a diet where the natural food has been replaced by highly processed foodstuffs have consistently shown increased aggressive behaviour.

The classic example is that of an American who was allergic to a specific red wine. He went out to dinner one evening, drank some of this wine, then stood up and shot several people. He was, of course, arrested, but denied intending to shoot those people. He was hospitalised and tested by being given various drinks disguised as red wine. One day, they gave him wine from the very same bottle. He lost control and had to be restrained. His reaction was real.

Our foods and environment, along with our immune responses to them, could have more to do with our behavioural as well as our medical problems than we realise. A lot more research needs to be done, but results to date look promising. The trouble is, it is a lot easier to tell a person to take a pill or two every day than it is to tell them to eliminate their favourite foods from their diet and to expect them to stick to it.

Alcoholism

Our tolerance of alcohol varies from individual to individual, but even the complete teetotaller has to cope with alcohol, and gets through roughly two measures of alcohol per day, though it never passes their lips (a measure of alcohol is equivalent to a glass of wine or half a pint of beer). Alcohol is made in all of us by the bugs that live in our gut and ferment our food; and people on a high sugar and refined food diet, and those with yeast infections in the gut, make more alcohol than the rest of the population.

The liver deals with the alcohol, releasing a zinc-dependent enzyme which renders it harmless. In a zinc-sufficient person with normal liver function one measure of alcohol is dealt with in roughly half an hour. When alcohol intake exceeds the body's ability to process it we get light-headed and then drunk.

Studies done with alcoholics now show that they often have sensitivities to wheat, corn, rye, malt, sugar or yeast. People without sensitivities to these related foods are less likely to become addicted to alcohol, even though they may drink a lot more than those who are.

Fits and heart problems

Ingestion of or exposure to food or chemical allergens can bring on fits, irregular heartbeats, high blood pressure, chest pains and blood clots. Research is still relatively new and incomplete in this area, but there is the possibility that some strokes and heart-related problems could be avoided if only we could recognise our food and chemical sensitivities, deficiencies and excesses.

Inflammatory bowel diseases

Inflammatory bowel diseases like Crohn's disease and ulcerative colitis are often blamed on food sensitivities, but exclusive diets should not be undertaken without professional guidance, as people with gut problems are often already very nutrient deficient due to the inability of the gut to digest and absorb normally. Antibodies to cows' milk and salicylates are often found in someone with ulcerative colitis, but avoiding foods containing these does not always bring relief. Supplements (of zinc in particular) are often required.

Coeliac disease is a sensitivity to gluten (found in wheat and some other cereals), but may well include a sensitivity to the rest of the grains as well.

Arthritis

Arthritis comes in various different forms. It is really a term which covers several conditions that have similar effects on the joints, but there is no definite single cause. Treatment, likewise, varies and what may be a miracle cure for one person can have no effect at all on another.

Food and chemical allergies have been cited as major offenders in many cases of rheumatoid arthritis, with remarkable claims from people confined to wheelchairs who were able to get up and walk after eliminating certain foods like red meat or perhaps dairy products, wheat, tea or coffee from the diet. These foods have also been labelled as aggravators in cases of osteoarthritis. It should be mentioned that it is usually one or two of these major risk foods that are a problem and they vary from person to person. Exclusion diets will be considered in the next chapter, but they can be dangerous on a self-help basis if too much is left out.

Anti-inflammatory drugs are often prescribed to reduce the pain and swelling in arthritis, but they do nothing to make the disease any better. Dietary therapy can sometimes have an effect equal to, if not better than, these drugs. Zinc and copper are very important in reducing inflammation, but they need to be in balance, as they work together with manganese. If the balance of these three is right, inflammation is minimised. If they are out of balance, the pain increases. A copper bracelet seems to work very well for some arthritics, but others get an aggravation of symptoms or no effect at all as a result of wearing one. Probably the acidity of the skin dissolves small amounts of copper, which are then absorbed. If the patient has a low copper status, then additional copper brings relief. If, however, the copper is already high in this person and the zinc is low, there could be aggravation. This type of person may get relief from zinc supplementation, although the dose will be dependent on the individual. The fatty acids are the building blocks of fats, just as amino acids are the building blocks of proteins. We can synthesise most of the fatty acids we need, but there are three - arachidonic, linoleic and alpha-linolenic acids - that we are unable to manufacture and that are needed for a wide range of functions. We therefore have to ensure that these are provided in the diet. But that is not all; we also have to ensure that we receive these EFA's (essential fatty acids) in the right proportions. In particular, if the balance is tipped in favour of arachidonic acid, it appears to promote the production of substances called leukotrienes in the mast cells - and leukotrienes are many times more inflammatory than histamine. A reduction in the intake of saturated fats and an increased intake of the unprocessed polyunsaturates, particularly cold-pressed safflower oil, cod liver oil and EPA (eicosapentaenoic acid, a derivative of alpha-linolenic acid, and available as a supplement), swings the balance away from arachidonic acid and may well be of benefit in arthritis.

Poor mineral absorption is also often a contributory factor in arthritis. Diets that include tea and coffee, or bran with everything, should be avoided as these deplete vitamin and mineral absorption. A balanced supplement may be necessary, but make sure you consult someone who knows what they are doing, as you will be using nutritional supplements like drugs. For example, iron supplements should not be taken by anyone with any inflammatory condition such as arthritis.

9

ALLERGY TESTS - ARE THEY WORTH IT?

The classic definition of an allergy is 'any idiosyncratic reaction where the immune system is clearly involved'. The immune system, which is the body's defence system, has the ability to produce 'markers' for substances it doesn't like. The classic marker is an antibody called IgE (immunoglobulin type E). These attach themselves to 'mast cells' in the body. When the offending allergen complexes with its specific IgE antibody, the IgE molecule triggers the mast cell to release granules containing histamine and other chemicals that cause the symptoms of classic allergy - skin rashes, hayfever, rhinitis, sinusitis, asthma and eczema. Severe food allergies to, for example, shellfish or peanuts, cause immediate gastrointestinal upsets or swelling in the face or throat. All these reaction are immediate, severe inflammatory reactions and are known as Type 1 allergic reactions.

Testing for type 1 allergy - IgE based

Skin prick test

This test involves putting a drop of the allergen (e.g. pollen) on the skin and scratching or pricking the skin to allow the allergen to enter the body. If local inflammation occurs then the test is positive.

Advantages: Good for skin related allergies. Moderate for inhalant allergies.

Disadvantages: Poor for food allergies. Will fail to pick up non IgE mediated allergy, has a poor success rate with IgE based food allergy, and may fail to pick up localised allergic reactions (for example, a person may have localised IgE antibodies to pollen in the nasal passages and not on the skin).

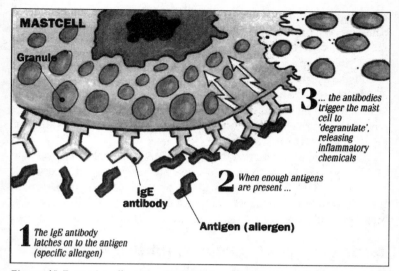

Figure of IgE, meeting allergen, and triggering mast cell to degranulate, causing reaction.

Intradermal test

This test involves injecting a small quantity of the suspect food under the skin in the hope that this more 'direct' contact may pick up food allergies better. It is still detecting IgE mediated reactions.

Advantages: It seems to produce better results than the skin prick test for food allergies and has an associated treatment involving finding the dilution of the allergen that doesn't cause a reaction. The person then takes this dilution, often as drops, on a regular basis to 'immunise' themselves from the allergen.

Disadvantages: Same as for skin prick tests.

RAST type tests

The RAST (radioallergosorbent test) involves taking a blood sample. The blood is then spun to separate red blood cells from the serum, which is rich where IgE antibodies are found. The serum is then put on top of specially prepared sample of potential allergens (extracts of food etc.). If the serum contains IgE to that substance it makes a complex. Another substance, called anti-IgE, is then introduced and sticks to any IgE that has complexed with the test substances. This anti-IgE is marked, either coloured or radioactive, and the severity of the colouration or radioactivity of each substance tested determines the level of IgE sensitivity. There are many variations of this basic method of testing IgE sensitivity which are broadly speaking comparable.

Advantages: It is the most accurate test for IgE based allergies and is more likely to pick up food allergies than skin tests. The person doesn't have to experience reactions nor go through the sometimes lengthy and painful procedure of skin testing.

Disadvantages: It is limited to IgE based reactions. A small percentage of IgE reactions do not show up because the reaction is localised (e.g. a food causing an IgE reaction only in the gut, or pollen only producing a reaction in the air passages) and produces no response in the blood. Many food allergies are not IgE based and therefore won't be identified.

Testing for type 3 allergy - probably IgG based

Cytotoxic tests

Cytotoxic tests involve introducing white blood cells to allergens and observing the response. The classic cytotoxic test involves a blood sample being taken, from which is isolated the white blood cells called neutrophils. These have the job of 'eating up' immune complexes in the

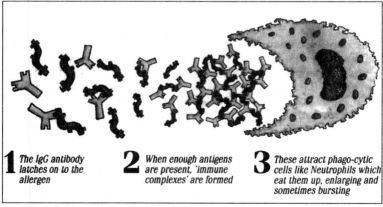

1 The IgG antibody latches on to the allergen

2 When enough antigens are present, 'immune complexes' are formed

3 These attract phago-cytic cells like Neutrophils which eat them up, enlarging and sometimes bursting

Figure of IgG complexes attracting neutrophil

body that are the result of hostile reactions. They are, if you like, vacuum cleaners for anything labelled as dirt, which is normally an invading protein. The neutrophils are exposed to the potential allergen and left to incubate for 90 minutes. The result is viewed under a microscope. If the neutrophil has reacted, it first becomes more rounded, then produces bubbles as it releases chemical weaponry to fight the invader and, in a severe reaction, bursts leaving an empty 'ghost cell'. These levels of reaction are graded to give a level of severity in the report.

Advantages: It is not limited to IgE responses and measures actual reactions of the body's immune system to particular substances.

Disadvantages: The test is dependent on the skill of the laboratory technician and their judgement regarding the grading of reactions. Cytotoxic tests are also more likely to show reactions to foods eaten most recently, since these foods may have primed the immune system to react. A dairy allergic who never has dairy may come up negative. Some recommend fasting for 12 hours before the blood sample is taken to minimise this effect. Generally, this test is considered by some to be 50-70% reliable.

Automated cytotoxic tests

Cytotoxic tests are very labour intensive and because of this and the fact that the results depend on the skill of the technician, allergists are investigating ways of standardising and automating the testing procedure. An example of this is the Nutron test which works on a similar principle to a cytotoxic test. Once the blood sample has been incubated with the potential allergen, an automatic haemotology unit 'interrogates' the cells through direct current, radio frequency changes and changes in size and number. If, after incubation there are a reduced number, this indicates that some have burst or, in immunospeak, the neutrophils have degranulated. The changes are analysed by a computer to give a read out on suspect foods and degrees of reaction. Theoretically results should be comparable to cytotoxic tests. No comparative tests have been carried out to my knowledge.

Advantages: The measuring process is automated and should, therefore, be more reproducible.

Disadvantages: To date this method is new and not yet proven. Anecdotal reports vary.

ELISA IgG food sensitivity tests

ELISA stands for 'Enzyme Linked Immuno Sorbent Assay' and is a well proven process used, for example, for detecting HIV positivity. In this case the technology is used to detect IgG positivity and the degree of reaction. The potential allergen has to be very carefully prepared into 'plates', and then the patient's serum is introduced to it. If there is an IgG reaction to the food the IgG antibody in the serum combines with the allergen on the plate. After an incubation time of some hours, water plus an enzyme is added, which colours the antibody-allergen complexes. The more antibody-allergen complexes there are the more coloured the sample becomes. This is analysed by computer to produce a graded scale of reaction to each food. The greater the reaction, the greater the sensitivity.

Advantages: The laboratory we investigated (Immuno Laboratories) reported the highest quality and reproducibility controls. Firstly, they had developed standard serum and tested each 'allergen plate' to ensure that the prepared plates would produce the same reactions. Secondly, they analysed split samples of serum every week to check they produced the same results, which they did. So the reproducibility was good. Two pilot studies and anecdotal reports have given good results in reducing symptoms by avoiding foods that test positive.This is a specific and well controlled qualitative IgG sensitive test.

Disadvantages: Apart from the debate as to the relevance of IgG testing, there is no disadvantage to this test other than the price.

The emerging view now is that most food allergies and intolerances, diplomatically called by some 'idiosyncratic' reactions, are not IgE based. There is a new school of thought and a new generation of allergy tests, designed to detect intolerances not based on IgE antibody reactions, but probably involving another marker, known as IgG. According to Dr James Braly, director of Immuno Laboratories, which developed the IgG ELISA test, "Food allergy is not rare, nor are the effects limited to the air passages, the skin and digestive tract. Most food allergies are delayed reactions, taking anywhere from an hour to three days to show themselves, and are therefore much harder to detect. Delayed food allergy appears to be simply the inability of your digestive tract to prevent large quantities of partially digested and undigested food from entering the bloodstream."

This is not a new idea. Since the 1950's pioneering allergists such as Dr Theron Randolph, Herbert Rinkel, Dr Arthur Coca, and, more recently, Dr William Philpott and Dr Marshall Mandel have written about delayed sensitivities causing far-reaching effects on all systems of the body. These were the 'heretics' of classic allergy theory, however their ideas are now being proven right with advances in scientific methods for determining other types of immune reactions.

IgG antibodies were first discovered in the 1960's and are still considered reasonably irrelevant by some conventional allergists The problem, say the critics, is that most people have many IgG based reactions to foods without apparently suffering from allergies. The IgG antibodies may serve as 'tags' but don't initiate a reaction. However, say the advocates, a large build-up of IgG antibodies to a particular food indicates a chronic long-term sensitivity, or food intolerance. It is now well established that many, if not the majority of food intolerances do not produce immediate symptoms, but have a delayed, accumulative effect. This, of course, makes them hard to detect by observation. Dr Hill, researching in Australia, found that the majority of food sensitive children reacted after 2 or more hours to foods. In contrast IgE reactions are immediate, suggesting that a build up of IgG antibodies may be a primary factor in food sensitivity.

According to Dr Jonathan Brostoff, consultant in medical immunology at the Middlesex Hospital Medical School, certain ingested substances can cause the release of histamine and invoke classical allergic symptoms without involving IgE. These include lectins (in peanuts), shellfish, tomatoes, pork, alcohol, chocolate, pineapple, papaya, buckwheat, sunflower, mango and mustard. He also thinks it is possible that undigested proteins could directly affect mast cells which contain histamine, in the gut, causing the classic symptoms of allergy.

One common reaction, known as Type 3 allergy, is said to occur when there is a substantial production of antibodies (mainly IgG) in response to an allergen in the blood. This results in immune complexes. "It is the sheer weight of numbers that causes a problem," says Brostoff. "These immune complexes are like litter going round in the bloodstream." The litter is cleaned up by cells, principally neutrophils, that act like vacuum cleaners. Cytotoxic allergy tests are designed to measure changes in number, size and activity of neutrophils when exposed to certain foods, to determine possible food allergies.

How IgG and IgE antibodies relate is another area of debate. Allergy specialist Dr Braly has seen a number of patients who have both an immediate and delayed reaction to a food, suggesting a link between the immediate short-term IgE type reaction and the delayed IgG reaction. Dr Anders Hoy from Denmark suspects that long-term build up of IgG to a particular food might switch to an IgE type sensitivity, causing immediate allergic response.

IgG allergy testing - the new generation?

The first type of tests to move away from measuring immediate IgE reactions were the 'cytotoxic' tests, which means 'toxic to cells'. These tests observe changes to immune cells called neutrophils which come along and clean up 'immune complexes' caused by antibody-antigen reactions. Cytotoxic tests are thought to reflect IgG sensitivity.

The state-of-the-art for measuring IgG sensitivity is a relatively new technique, developed over the last eight years, involving a method known as ELISA. ELISA testing for IgG sensitivity claims more reproducible and reliable results than cytotoxic testing, and indeed samples tested by both methods have little agreement in results. One possibility is that these tests measure different types of reactions. Another is that one or more of the tests is unreliable.

Allergy or indigestion?

Dr Hoy, who is a convert to the new ELISA IgG testing, believes that 'healthy' foods cause allergic reaction because they are not properly digested. "If food is not broken down into small molecules you start producing IgG antibodies. The immune cells have to work hard to produce masses of IgGs, reducing the immune system's capacity for fighting infection." says Hoy, who has observed that people with pronounced IgG reactions produce little stomach acid, which would lead to poor digestion and a greater chance of allergy. Whether this is a cause or effect of allergy isn't clear, however, for many allergy sufferers low hydrochloric acid production is part of the picture.

Both Dr Hoy and Dr Braly prescribe the same remedy - avoid foods that provoke an IgG reaction to lessen the load on the immune system, and then focus on improving digestion. Dr Braly has found zinc deficiency to be extremely common among allergy sufferers. Zinc is not only needed to digest all protein, it's also essential for the production of hydrochloric acid in the stomach. Certain foods, he says, are inherently difficult to digest, the worst being gluten in wheat, and bovine serum in dairy products. Wheat and dairy are Britain's top two allergy provoking foods.

He also suspects that many allergy sufferers may have excessively 'leaky' gut walls, allowing undigested proteins to enter the blood and cause reactions. Consumption of alcohol, frequent use of aspirin, deficiency in essential fatty acids or a gastrointestinal infection or infestation such as candidiasis are all possible contributors to leaky gut syndrome that need to be corrected to reduce a person's sensitivity to foods.

Cross-reaction

Another contributor to food sensitivity is exposure to inhalants that provoke a reaction. For example, it is well known that, when the pollen count in high more people suffer from hayfever in polluted areas than in rural areas despite lower pollen counts in cities. It is thought that exposure to exhaust fumes makes a pollen-allergic more sensitive. Whether this is simply because their immune system is weakened from dealing with the pollution and therefore less able to cope with the additional pollen insult, or due to some kind of 'cross-reaction' is not known. In the US, where ragweed sensitivity is common, a cross-reaction with bananas has been reported. In other words, one sensitivity sensitises you to another. A similar cross-reaction may occur with pollen, wheat and milk for hayfever sufferers.

The emerging view, shared by an increasing number of allergy specialists is that food sensitivity is a multi-factorial phenomenon possibly involving poor nutrition, pollution, digestive problems and over-exposure to certain foods. Removing the foods may help the immune system to recover, but other factors need to be dealt with in order to have a major impact on long-term food intolerance.

How long to avoid?

Just how long allergens have to be avoided is another open-ended question. Foods that invoke an IgE type, immediate and pronounced reaction may need to be avoided for life. The 'memory' of IgE antibodies is long-term. In contrast, B-cells that produce IgG antibodies have a half-life of six weeks. That means that there are half as many six weeks later. The 'memory' of these antibodies is short-term and, within six months, there is unlikely to be any residual 'memory' of reaction to a food that's been avoided. While a six month avoidance may be ideal, Hoy and Braly report good results after as little as a month. Another option, after a strict one month avoidance, is to 'rotate' foods so that an IgG sensitive food is only eaten every 4 days. This reduces the build up of allergen-antibody complexes and reduces the chances of symptoms of intolerance. Foods such as wheat and milk which are, by their nature, difficult to digest, are probably best avoided as much as possible.

Which test is best?

Testing allergy tests is notoriously difficult and falls into three stages - testing reproducibility, testing reliability, testing usefulness.

Any allergy test should have proven reproducibility. That is, split samples taken at the same time by the same method should produce the same result. Then there is the question of day to day reliability. If a test produces substantially different results from day to day then how useful is the information? One cannot assume that, because something happens to the neutrophils during a lab test, that the person will experience symptoms. If these reactions happen to whatever was eaten last then what does the patient do? Avoid all foods? Finally, there is the big question. How useful is the test? Does avoidance of the identified allergens improve health, and result in less symptoms of ill-health? This is where it gets tricky. Let's suppose you have twenty people tested, each of which tests positive to ten foods. You could have them avoid those ten foods and see if their health improves. Or you could take each food, have the person avoid it, then reintroduce it and record symptoms. This is very complex and even this kind of testing is not 'double-blind'. Consequently, few worthwhile trials have been carried out, especially on the more recently developed testing methods. Practitioners rely on the results they achieve with patients.

10

FOOD SENSITIVITIES AND SLIMMING

A girl came to see me for nutritional advice. She looked dreadful, a sunken wreck. She was eating peanuts - that was all, nothing but peanuts. She believed that she was allergic to various different foods and had been eliminating them one by one. By the time she came to see me she had given up everything except peanuts. A doctor from the eating disorder clinic at the Bristol Royal Infirmary confirmed that she was seeing other people doing the same sort of thing. It cannot be stressed enough that if you are slimming, or if you are trying to detect foods to which you are allergic, the more your restrict the variety of foods which you eat, the less balanced your diet is likely to be.

If you are slimming, 1,000 calories, 4,200 joules or 4.2 kilojoules per day should be the absolute minimum, and these calories must be carefully selected to give the range of nutrients needed. Medical supervision is needed for anything less, and will probably be advised even at this level in many cases where there are additional health problems.

To detect food allergies only one or two food groups should be tested at a time. If there are multiple allergies, professional supervision is needed to make sure that nutrients are replaced in some other form.

Food and chemical sensitivities

Symptoms of food and chemical sensitivities are similar; indeed, the two often go hand in hand. For example, you may have no problem eating an organic apple or lettuce, but go into a spin after eating those that have been sprayed. If you find that you do have a reaction to a fruit, vegetable or grain, it is worth experimenting with the organic form just to make sure that it is not a reaction to a chemical used on the food.

Recent research has certainly shown that we can be allergic to, or become allergic to, everyday foods. Very often it is the foods that we have become addicted to and eat every day that cause the problems; hence the most common foods, such as wheat, eggs, sugar, milk and dairy produce, meat, tea and coffee, tend to the ones that most often cause problems. We are not all sensitive to the same foods; each of us is different.

Symptoms of sensitivities

Initial symptoms of food sensitivities may be vague, even mild, but they can change enigmatically or get more persistent as life continues. Like alcohol and drugs, a food or chemical can become addictive and can eventually cause more serious symptoms. It first gives an uplifting sensation and creates a desire for it, but it also has its hangover - the depressed or low reactions, some of which are listed below:
• Skin reactions can include eczema, itching patches, dryness, hives.
• Head reactions can include headaches, migraines; dizziness; fear of heights; unreal sensations like floating or being detached; ringing or fluid in the ears; earache; sensitivity to light, dull itchy eyes, watery eyes; emotional instability, crying or edgy laughter; frequent throat clearing or cough, rhinitis, voice irregularities.
• Chest symptoms can include bronchitis, breathing difficulties; irregular or pronounced heart beat; high blood pressure.
• Gut and trunk problems can include stomachache or swelling; constipation or diarrhoea; indigestion, nausea, vomiting; water retention, frequency of urination, bedwetting, especially in children allergic to coloured lollies or drinks.
• Muscle and joint pains can include vague and perhaps mobile aches and pains; swelling of joints; muscle spasms; unusual weakness, progressing later into rheumatism or arthritis.
• General symptoms can include poor concentration, inability to think clearly; lack of energy; irritability or moodiness, perhaps progressing to depression and despair.

Preventing sensitivity

The most desirable choice is to prevent sensitivity occurring, but it requires willpower. These suggestions help prevent further problems:
• Eat raw foods before cooked food. When we eat, white blood cells line up along the gut wall, and it seems that raw food does not cause destruction of these white blood cells as much as cooked food. The

French idea of crudités before a meal is a good habit to get into, and is also quite slimming.

• Avoid becoming addicted to any food by ensuring you don't eat the same item or items of food every day. If you are in good health and are not knowingly suffering from any allergy symptoms, one week in every ten without one's 'fix' may well be enough to prevent addiction. Milk is a common food to which we may become addicted if we suffer with a leaky gut because it is drunk in tea or coffee, providing little injections of it throughout the day, every day. Wheat, too, is a national addiction. Although we may think we have a varied diet, it is often only the added flavours and colours and the change of texture that is different. Bread, buns, cakes, pastries, pies, pasties, quiches, pizzas, batter, biscuits and breakfast cereals all contain wheat. It is, in fact, quite difficult to eliminate wheat entirely from the diet, because wheat is hidden in some form in many foods. There are many cereal grains that we could eat instead of wheat, and using them as part of the regular diet would improve our nutrition in more ways than one.

• Have a very varied diet using, as far as possible, fruits, vegetables and fish in their seasons. It is now possible to buy some foods, strawberries for example, nearly all year round; but, while strawberries are delicious, it is very easy to get an allergic reaction from them. So enjoy them whilst they are in season and then leave them alone for a while. Never narrow foods down to a monotonous daily routine.

• Use wholefoods rather than highly processed and chemically treated foods where possible.

Sensitivity reactions of some foods

Stimulants

Some sufferers can easily become addicted to stimulants like tea, coffee, alcohol, nicotine, sugar or simply overbreathing. When an allergen enters the stomach, it cause a war, and histamine is released. This, in turn, causes more biochemicals to be released from the stomach and the whole body, including the brain, gets a flood of these. The brain reacts to the chemical stimulation and the result is a 'high' feeling which is easy and pleasant to become addicted to.

Nuts

To the immune system, all nuts are similar and, having developed an allergy to one, it is easy to do the same for another. Nuts are the biggest seeds and in very sensitive people cause the tongue and throat to swell. Chocolate is a form of nut and so should be included in this category. Arthritics are often particularly sensitive to nuts and chocolate. It is unfortunate, as nuts are nutrient-packed foods, but it is necessary to rotate them in the diet.

Milk

It is possible to have an allergic reaction to cold milk but not to hot milk; this is due to an allergen which is destroyed on heating. This means that you may be able to drink milk which has been boiled.

A beef allergy does not have to go with a milk allergy, and cheeses have many different allergens in them unrelated to milk. So a cheese allergy does not necessarily rule out milk. And a milk allergic may well be able to eat butter, as milk fat and protein are different antigenically.

Fish

People allergic to bony fish (herring, mackerel, cod, haddock) may not be allergic to cartilaginous fish such as skate, ray, shark and dogfish, as the antigen is different. Similarly, the jointed and mollusc shellfish have different antigens. Shellfish are especially well known for causing allergies as they have copper-containing enzyme systems and a substance called haemocyanin which is a very powerful antigen and makes a lot of people develop urticaria or be sick.

Fruit and Vegetables

Allergic reactions from these are often due to chemicals sprayed on to them, but they do carry antigens of their own. Raw carrots and raw celery have a common antigen to which a few people become sensitive, but this is destroyed on cooking, so these individuals can eat cooked but not raw carrots and celery. Orange peel and apple pips have antigens which can cause problems. Onions, leeks and garlic have strong-reacting antigens - often the stronger the taste, the stronger the antigen.

Yeast

Even the smell of bakers' yeast can set some people off, and they certainly cannot eat bread and other foods containing yeast.

Meat

Lamb is usually the least likely to cause an allergy problem. Pork is often a problem in asthmatics and beef in rheumatoid arthritics. Adults with eczema sometimes cannot eat meat at all without a reaction.

What happens in food allergy

Most people think that food is digested in the gut and is then absorbed into the bloodstream, but sometimes, it seems, incompletely digested food goes straight into the bloodstream. This is known as persorption, and happens more often in people with weak or damaged guts.

The immune soldiers in the bloodstream get rid of the undigested food, but in doing so they make antibodies to it, treating it as an antigen. This is often how food allergy starts. Once the antibodies are made to a food, the body is sensitised and makes more of them when that food is encountered next. The result is that antigen/antibody complexes are formed, some of which may go to the liver; but others are deposited in joint spaces where they activate neutrophils and release a powerful free radical called superoxide - hence the arthritis link with food sensitivities.

The worst way to deal with a food sensitivity is to have the offending food little and often, because there will then always be more antibody available than there is antigen. This causes antibody/antigen complexes to be formed, and the symptoms of food sensitivity result. A better way to deal with the problem is to have a lot of the offending food in one go, and then forget about it completely for a few days. The body only makes a small amount of antibody at any one time and if the food (the allergen) is in excess of the antibody, there are fewer antibody/antigen complexes formed and less reaction. This is called masking.

Technically the gut is a tunnel running right through the body, and nutrients have to pass from the inside of the tunnel into the body. The immune system mounts little reaction to substances in the gut, i.e. in the tunnel, but a response will invariably be invoked if anything foreign - non-self - gets into the body through a faulty tunnel wall, without being processed first. The major lymphoid tissue in the gut is the Peyer's patches in the intestines, but there appears to be no such tissue above the level of the waist. In this region the principal immunological agent is IgA; this has limited biological activity, and no memory - which is just as well, otherwise we would become irrevocably sensitised to each and every food we consumed, and would only be able to eat them once. IgA is very thymus dependent, and gives rise to the most common of the immunodeficiencies, affecting about one in 700 people. These individuals tend to suffer a higher risk of sinopulmonary and gastrointestinal infections and a greater incidence of food sensitivities.

Hypoallergenic foods

People in this country are very rarely allergic to sago (from the trunk of a palm tree). Similarly, tapioca is usually safe; it is only 2% protein and is derived from African cassava. There have been no reported cases of allergy to rhubarb.

Elimination diet

If you suspect a food, leave it out of the diet completely for a week. You have to be very strict about this; cutting down is suffering for nothing. If you suspect a sensitivity and wish to test for it, it is all or nothing at all. It also means that all canned or processed and packeted foods are out for that week, because you are never absolutely sure what is in them. If you are eliminating wheat, this means eliminating everything that may contain even a trace of wheat. It probably means not baking with wheat for the rest of the family, as you would be likely to get some wheat this way. Similarly, it is no use using wheat flour to roll out your oatcakes if you are testing for wheat sensitivity.

If you are addicted to the food you are eliminating, withdrawal symptoms will probably occur during the first three days. Sometimes these can be very violent. If this happens, it may be necessary to come off the food slowly before withdrawing it completely. If you are really this hooked, medical help may be needed in order to give it up. For most people, though, symptoms are unpleasant, but mild and bearable, and usually disappear by the fourth day.

Leave the food out of the diet for the rest of the week or perhaps longer. Then pick a convenient day, if there is such a thing, when it does not matter if you do not perform your best and reintroduce the offending food or beverage on an empty stomach. if there are not violent symptoms, take it several more times throughout the day - in fact, make a pig of yourself on it. If you are allergic to it you should start to feel ill!

It may be necessary to eliminate foods that cause a reaction for six months or so; if this is the case, it will be necessary to find other foods to provide the nutrients that would have been supplied. After this time, the food may be reintroduced into the diet, and if it does not then cause any ill effect, you can have it occasionally, but not on a daily basis.

Rotation diet

We could all do with a diet where all real foods are eaten in moderation and in rotation, but this is not easy. We all get into our little daily habits.

The best plan of action for people with multi-allergies is to separate the food groups, eating, for example, wheat on Monday, oats and no wheat at all on Tuesday, rice for Wednesday, and so on. Some experts say that a four-day rotation diet will do; others say a seven-day rotation is necessary. It is probably safer and easier to go for the seven day rotation, the idea being that any offending food is totally eliminated for six days. This six-day gap does not allow the body to build up an addiction to the food and, most importantly, it allows you to eat! If wheat causes aggravation, for example, it is possible to leave it out for several months as long as it is replaced by another grain. (Most people in Britain live on a restricted diet of only one or two grains anyway.) Be adventurous, give your immune system a treat and vary your grains.

Unsuccessful slimming

Dr Berger is a doctor, a psychiatrist and a specialist in bariatrics (the science of weight control). He himself was once an enormous 30 stone (420 lb or 190kg) and could not lose weight. He tried all of the methods then used for weight loss, but they only made him sicker. He delved into nutritional immunology and found a secret that worked for him and one that has apparently worked for more that 3,000 of his patients who between them lost 74,000 lb (34,000 kg) of extra fat.

He is of the opinion that food sensitivities prevent many people from losing weight. He therefore recommends detection and elimination or rotation of problem foods. After the sensitivities have been identified, supplements help to repair the damaged immune system and allow stored fat to be utilised properly. The best way to slim is slowly, as this way the skin and stomach gradually go back to their normal size and do not look baggy. Sudden shock weight-loss can lead to sever immune deficiency and can eventually perpetuate the fat cycle; in short, inappropriate dieting can make you fat.

Hints for People with Food Sensitivities

• Reduce the number of antigens if possible; that is to say, eliminate chemicals and, as far as possible, the foods to which you are very sensitive. At the same time be careful not to put the diet out of balance. (The book Dr Braly's Food Allergy and Nutrition Revolution will be useful.)

• Improve protein digestion by chewing food well and eating it separate from carbohydrates. In this way, whole proteins are less likely to pass through the gut wall into the body. (Food combining will help with this type of eating pattern.)

• Improve gut mucosal integrity with nutrients, in particular, zinc, pantothenic acid and beta-carotene.

• Reduce sugar and spices which aggravate gut membranes.

• Reduce animal fat consumption and increase the intake of linoleic acid.

• Increase the intake of antioxidants - vitamins E and C, beta-carotene, zinc, copper and manganese.

Conclusion

Food sensitivities, as we have seen, cause a vast range of physical, mental and emotional problems. Some people become addicted or develop eating disorders like bingeing, because the foods which cause the damage release beta-endorphins. These are brain chemicals that act a bit like opium; they give relief from pain and give a sensation of well-being; they control appetite, sexual desire and body temperature; but eventually they cause depression. Food can give us pleasure or cause us pain; it can make us fit or make us sick. There is a very strong link between our nutrition and the immune system.

Food allergy is not a simple disease. It is a condition of many causes, many mechanisms with no single cure. It must be remembered that most people do not have serious food allergies and most people should be able to eat and enjoy a wide variety of foods.

Part 3

BOOSTING YOUR IMMUNE POWER

11

THE HISTORY OF HEALING

The Ancient Greeks had a god and a goddess of healing. The god of healing was Aesculapius, and his staff with a snake coiled around it has been adopted by the medical profession. He stood for the more invasive, toxic procedures which needed to be used in emergency situations and which would equate with surgery, radiation therapy, chemotherapy and drug therapy today.

Hygeia, the goddess of health and beauty, stood for healing by gentle, natural means, using the five things that the body requires to live, ie. food, water, air, light and love. Even then, around 400 BC, healing was seen to take place from within. If invasive methods of treatment have to be used, eg. the amputation of a limb, the body still has to heal the wound.

Hippocrates, the Greek physician and author of around seventy books on all aspects of ancient medicine is famous for his saying, ' Let food be your medicine'. He believed in and saw the necessity for both forms of healing and is now known as,' the Father of Modern Medicine'. Ironically, although medical students take the Hippocratic Oath, they often pay little attention to food, bar recommending that elusive 'balanced diet'.

This book obviously only deals with improving our own ability to strengthen our own immune system, with the aim of minimising susceptibility to disease and increasing the ability to heal from within using natural methods. The guidelines and observations in this book are in no way intended to be prescriptive. We are all unique and will have different requirements at different stages of life, but we all share a common basis in physiology and biochemistry. Everyone needs to take some responsibility for their own learning, lifestyle and health and if we can learn to identify what our bodies need at any given moment in time, we can modify our lifestyles accordingly to keep them healthy.

There is no single formula that will work for everyone all of the time, the scales of health are continually changing throughout life, but it is never too early or too late to start improving your health and your life. We cannot avoid all of the threats to the immune system but we can lessen the load and so help to maintain that vital balance which could otherwise so easily tip those scales in favour of disease.

12

EXERCISE AND YOUR IMMUNE SYSTEM

D o you wake up most mornings, refreshed and full of enthusiasm for the day ahead? Do you go to work looking good and feeling good, with a smile on your face, or do you drag yourself there, clothes flung on in haste, wearing a harassed expression and facing the work, the people and the pressures with a certain amount of dread?

Does your body work well and painlessly or does it creak, groan and hurt when you ask it to do that little bit extra? Do you often feel depressed, lethargic, irritable or tense? Are headaches, backaches, PMT, allergies or infections frequent companions? Obviously none of us feels wonderful all of the time, but we should most of the time. It is the attitude with which we cope with problems that determines whether we make the most out of the problems and pleasures in life or whether life becomes a trial.

Most of us spend hours every day working to earn money with which to live. We also spend a considerable amount of time cleaning, maintaining and repairing our homes and possessions. Little thought and time, in comparison, is spent on cleaning, maintaining and repairing our bodies, even though we are stuck with the same model for all of our lives; there is no trading it in for one that looks better, feels better, works better and is generally in better condition!

Body lab

The body is a complex living laboratory. It has mental, emotional, social, physical and chemical needs which have to be provided for if it is to work efficiently and well. The immune system is responsible for the condition of this body and the thoughts and love, movement and light, air, water and food that we feed it will all affect this system and hence the body as a whole. The cleaner and better maintained we are, both inside and out, the longer we are liable to stay in good condition.

We function best when we feel in control of body and mind and the situations that we find ourselves in, when we have confidence in ourselves and our abilities, so set your aims and goals at an achievable level for you. Don't keep comparing yourself to others and try to reach their standards, all you would need is half a dozen friends, each with their own but different enviable strengths and you would be in overdrive trying to keep up. Maintain your own strengths, identify your weaker areas and decide where to improve.

It is relatively easy to spot a person who has this immune boosting control and confidence. They may not have great wealth or possessions, or whatever you regard as a sign of success but, they have a clear direction in life, a body that is held and moved with pride and ease, a charisma which is not necessarily dependent on expensive clothes nor obvious, inherited good looks. They smile genuine smiles with their eyes as well as their mouths, and speak and act with a quiet confidence. They are in control. Even when there are problems they can be relied upon to cope. They can accept their own role in life without constant grumbling and have a positive attitude, they enjoy life, most of the time.

How can you help your immune system

There are many ways in which we can help our immune system to stay fit and healthy, so reducing our susceptibility to premature ageing and disease. The master key for all of them is BALANCE. To be out of balance in any area is to tip the scales of life against us. For ease of discussion, we have to divide things up and even leave some things out, but it should be remembered that it is the person as a whole that counts and all of our systems are interrelated and dependent on one another for the healthy functioning of the whole.

The effect of exercise on the immune system

We have a network of tubes throughout our bodies called the lymphatic system. It is very similar to the blood system, but whereas the latter has the heart to keep the blood moving, the lymphatic system relies on muscular contractions throughout the body to keep the lymph moving along the lymphatic vessels. Lymph is heavier when it contains a lot of fat, so a high fat diet and not much exercise is a recipe for a stagnant, inefficient immune system. It is known that exercise alters the fat profile of the blood for the better. It also strengthens the heart, decreases the resting pulse rate and increases a sense of well-being by causing the production of hormone-like chemicals called endorphins.

Vigorous exercise also disperses corticosteroids produced during stress. If not dispersed, these cause the thymus and lymph nodes to shrink, and interferon and T-cell production to decrease. Exercise improves circulation, thus increasing both oxygen supply to tissues and toxic waste removal.

As the lymph contains a vast proportion of our immune army, it is obviously important to keep it on the move. The human body was designed to move and too much sitting watching TV needs to be balanced with sufficient exercise to keep us at a whole and our immune system in particular, active. It should also be remembered that too much exercise, as in excessive training, can also suppress the immune system. Everybody is different and requires different levels of exercise. The golden rules are: to warm up slowly, to stop if it hurts and try again later, to exercise little and often to start with, and to improve the standard gradually.

With our increased technology and division of labour our purity of movement is often destroyed. We have various joints, sets of muscles and organs that were designed to be used but many of us now follow a sedentary lifestyle, both at work and at home. We go from home to the car; to the office and back to the car; to the television set and then to bed. This is a very restricting movement and not at all what we were intended to do. Paradoxically this sort of existence can make us feel very tired, and even less inclined to do exercise.

We need a balance in our movement, as in all other things. People these days can suffer from repetitive strain injury, caused by too much use of the pressure on certain muscles - usually the fingers and wrists, yet the same people often suffer from stiff and degenerating joints, simply because they do not use most of them enough; they are constantly sitting cramped up and inactive, using little apart from their keyboard fingers.

The very mention of exercise often increases the desire to put your feet up and have a cup of tea, but we need to move. Most of us are not aiming at top athlete training or maximum physical capacity, all we want to do is to move easily and without pain for as much of our lives as possible and so be able to enjoy life to the full. This means avoiding pollution of movement, and restoring the purity of movement that we are all capable of achieving. What can we do?

General stamina

Firstly we need to consider those vital internal organs such as the heart and lungs. How flexible and capable are they? How well do they cope with doing that little bit extra? We want to be able to run up the stairs or after the children without feeling out of breath.

Some form of regular exercise (and by that I mean weekly or preferably daily, not yearly) that increases the heart beat and breathing to a comfortable, but nevertheless, higher level, is required here. Walking briskly for half an hour is fine; if you feel more energetic, cycling, swimming, skipping, jogging, racket sports, or aerobic exercise are also suitable.

This form of exercise will not only improve the heart and lungs; it will also improve general stamina, the ability to last without flagging in normal daily life. Although swimming is good for the heart, lungs and general stamina, it does not help to retain bone density, so it is not good as the only form of exercise if you are past middle age, as it does not help in preventing osteoporosis. A good form of exercise if you really don't have a lot of time is skipping. It increases heart and breathing rate and is a very good load bearing exercise which has been proven to be good in preventing osteoporosis. It's cheap, doesn't take a lot of room and you can stop or start whenever you need to. Yoga and t'ai chi, although not 'aerobic' as such, have been shown to boost immunity and have many overall health benefits.

Breathing

The lungs age quite rapidly compared to other organs, usually through loss of capacity, which is in turn brought about by lack of use. Breathing deeply and properly is vitally important to stop this unnecessary premature degeneration. With loss of lung capacity comes inefficient and insufficient carriage of oxygen to other parts of the body, which in turn can increase the risk of cancer (cancer cells switch to an anaerobic i.e.

without oxygen, form of respiration to obtain their energy). It can also decrease powers of concentration and efficiency, as well as increase feelings of depression.

For those who are less mobile, singing or playing a wind instrument, or even deep and varied breathing can improve this situation.

Aerobic exercise

A sedentary lifestyle, possibly combined with poor posture, bad work position and tension, increases the necessity for part of the body to be devoted to some form of vigorous exercise as long as you don't overdo it.

Your ideal exercising pulse rate is between 60% and 80% of 220 minus your age. So, if you're 40 years old that's 180 x 60% = 108 and 180 x 80% = 144. So your ideal pulse rate during exercise would be between 108 and 144 beats per minute. This is a good guide; it makes sure you do enough exercise to do some good, but not so much as to yourself harm. As your fitness improves, so your resting pulse rate should go down.

Too much aerobic exercise, however, can both depress immunity and increase the risk of upper respiratory infections. So, once again, the key is balance.

Flexibility

Next we need to feel that we are supple, that we can bend but not break. When we have to sit in a fixed position for long periods of time, muscles can shorten and stiffen, and the flow of lymph around the body slows down. This causes various aches and pains, particularly in the neck. The lymph cleans up toxins and fights bugs less efficiently, as it needs muscular movement to push it around.

To be flexible we need to keep all the joints well oiled and mobile. Stretching and bending exercises are necessary to achieve this degree of movement. Massage can also help, especially for those that cannot move easily. Massage of course, also helps, with relaxation and the feelings of well being associated with touch; it is an excellent family activity, which can decrease strain and tension. You can even do it whilst watching the television if you are a TV addict.

Strength and tone

We require strength, not only to lift the children and to push and pull furniture or the car, but to hold our tummies in, to pump our blood and lymph around, and to look firm and in control of our muscles rather than appearing flabby. It is not necessary to go to regular weight training to achieve strength, although weight-lifting is good for this.

The aim is not to be a champion strong man, but to look firm, to feel fit and not weak, to prevent premature muscle degeneration and have the strength to do all of the necessary pulling, pushing and lifting with ease. Sit-ups and press-ups are good for increasing strength, as are cycling and rowing.

Moving naturally

In daily life, try to move naturally more often. Play with the children instead of just organising them; garden more often, or take up some other active hobby. If you don't want a dog, take the children, a friend or even just take yourself for a walk. Carry the groceries of course, unless you shop once a week and have an unmanageable amount. Take the stairs rather than the lift or elevator, and perhaps do some of the more strenuous DIY jobs by hand sometimes.

Remember that the way you breathe and the way you sit, stand or lift are vital. Do them the right way and you improve your condition; do them the wrong way and you could end up flat on your back for weeks. Try to find all of your muscles, and use them all sometimes. Many muscles can be exercised whilst we do mundane things; you can relax and contract stomach muscles, repeatedly raise yourself on your tiptoe and lower yourself again, and even contract and relax the female pelvic floor whilst standing washing up or peeling the vegetables.

If you are going to sit and watch TV after a relatively sedentary day, simple stretching and bending exercises can be done in the comfort of your own chair. If you really need to sit and relax, however, at least sit properly so you do not crush your stomach and give yourself indigestion, or cross your legs and impair circulation, or slouch and strain your back.

The way you move throughout your life says a lot about how you are and how you will be in the years to come.

Advantages of movement

Depending on age, weight, etc., movement that increases the heart beat sufficiently for around 20 minutes per day would be extremely valuable in:

• Either maintaining normal or reducing high blood pressure.
• Either maintaining a low or reducing a high resting pulse rate.
• Changing the fat profile of the blood in favour of less harmful fats.
• Maintaining normal body weight and muscle tone
• Increasing the sense of well being and improving self image.
• Keeping the immune army on the move; remember it is muscular contraction which keeps the lymph moving and allows transport of immune soldiers.
• Increasing energy levels.
• Dispersing toxins which build up in a sedentary body.
• Strengthening bones (minerals come out of bones whilst sleeping or if we have a sedentary lifestyle). Exercise helps to deposit minerals in the bone bank.

Relaxing

On top of this general all-round movement, we need relaxation and sound sleep.

Relaxation is as important as movement, but not if you slump into an ill-fitting chair which will strain the spine, cause constriction of blood flow (a badly positioned bar or crossed legs or leaning on an arm), crunch up body organs (especially the stomach and intestines, putting an end to digestion and leaving partially digested food to cause gas, pain, indigestion and constipation) and prevent lymph movement.

We spend about twenty years of our lives sleeping, and it's deprivation for twenty days would bring about death. Blood pressure, pulse rate, temperature and metabolic rate fall during sleep. Sweat production increases, so ridding the body of toxins accumulated during the day. Delta sleep (stages 3 & 4) is very important for immune function as it is during this stage that the pituitary gland steps up production of growth hormone, which in turn stimulates the thymus gland, so essential for T cell activity.

13

POSITIVE THINKING

J ust as we are what we eat, drink and breathe, so we are what we think. Our minds and personalities are built up out of the thoughts with which they are fed and on which they dwell. It is as easy to pollute the mind as it is to pollute the air, food and water. For example, people who, often without realising it, cultivate unhealthy, negative and distressing thoughts are generally more prone to mental and physical illness than those who dwell on the happier, more positive thoughts. Polluted thinking can be just as devastating to the body as environmental pollution. Morbid, frightening, distressful, hateful, helpless and unhappy thoughts can be just as toxic as alcohol, cigarettes and drugs when they are taken to excess. Fortunately, we do have some control over what we fill our minds with, and can choose the healthier options.

Life has many problems, so it is not always possible to be on top of the world. But it is not so much the problems as our attitudes toward them that determine whether we come through each stress or drown in our sorrows. It is all very well suggesting changing thought patterns to happier thoughts, but quite another thing to do it if you have suffered bereavement or are desperately worried about a job loss, financial problems or ill health. Such suggestions must never the less be made because, unless the thought is actually put in to a depressed person's head, they are unlikely to think of it themselves. It often takes a determined effort to balance upsetting thoughts with more pleasant ones, and it can be harder than changing your diet. What can we do?

Balance

We need to be able to balance whatever life throws at us with constructive thoughts and actions. Obviously we all have to cope with bereavements, disappointments and pain at various times - events that will make us unhappy. Indeed, it is necessary to feel unhappy when sad things happen; we would be very cold and uncaring individuals if we felt nothing at all. But although we need to feel sad, we should not dwell on these sad feelings all of the time. Life goes on and a balance has to be found.

Choice

Every day we have the choice: we can make the best of that day; we can do only what we have to do; or we can waste the day completely. The choice is always ours. It is a good idea, every day, to do something that you want to do opposed to that which you have to do; to smile; to be enthusiastic; to think beautiful thoughts for some of the time; even if you are being given a diet of problems. It is vital to believe in yourself, even if you are being put down. Opinion is, after all, only relative. So know and trust your own instincts and abilities and never lose your sense of humour.

Thought and the immune system

We know that changes in our thought patterns can bring about physical and emotional changes. When we are in love or happy we look and feel better than we do when we are depressed and miserable. With positive thinking we can increase our white blood cell count and improve the immune system and resistance to infection. Depression brings about the reverse. Many studies have shown decreased immune function in states of depression. While some people can visualise themselves well and become well, sometimes even to the extent of shrinking tumours, others can make themselves sick with depressive thoughts.

It has also been shown that we can increase the size of the thymus and even the number of T lymphocytes by the way we think. Pollution of the mind can thus cause very real physical and emotional problems. So it is that a continual diet of violent videos, for example, or hateful thoughts, is not to be encouraged. Even thinking of nothing very much can alter the personality, making it boring, bored, and often lazy. Habitual negative thoughts can bring about addiction and anti-social behaviour. The mind needs exercise; creative daydreaming is not a waste of time, and the more beautiful the thoughts that can be taken in or created, the more pleasure can be brought by recalling these at a later date.

Look for and recognise polluted thoughts, and replace them

whereever possible. Make sure that you are in control of your thoughts and your life and that they are not controlling you. At least think about it!

Life is not always fair, painless and trouble free and there is little doubt from the scientific literature that major life stresses deplete immunity. Yet it is only natural that we feel sad or depressed sometimes, but the good news is that the body caters for that as well. Crying relieves tension and washes away toxic chemicals produced by our distress. On analysis, it has been found that tears caused by peeling onions are little more than salt and water compared to the complex chemical cocktail produced when tears are the result of stress. Exercise, also, increases the body's own pick-me-ups, the endorphins, to help put us back in balance. The fastest and most effective way to change your life is to change your attitude. A hardening of the attitudes can be as destructive as a hardening of the arteries, but it is reversible if you want it to be.

Thought vitamins

Below are a few useful 'thought vitamins ' that may help in achieving a more positive attitude to life.

• Laugh at least once a day. It is good for the digestion as well as your emotional well being. Cultivate a sense of humour.
• Enthusiasm gives you energy, boredom makes you tired.
• If you decide to do something, do it wholeheartedly not halfheartedly.
• Posture conveys your attitude to others. Feel tall, walk tall. Slouch and everyone knows that you can't be bothered.
• Happiness and confidence causes secretions of endorphins in the body which further increase our feelings of well being, and boost immunity.
• We all make mistakes. That's how we learn.
• Hard work is good for you as long as you enjoy it.
• Sadness is necessary sometimes, but don't dwell on for too long.
• Blows to life will sometimes knock you down. That is no reason to crawl for ever. Get up and go in another direction, or just try again.
• An accumulation of small difficulties can sometime sap more of your energy than one big problem. Be aware of small leaks and deal with them.
• Attitudes are more important than facts.
• When you get up in the morning you have two choices, to be happy or unhappy. Choose carefully.

- Set yourself goals you can reach. It is not a good idea to set yourself impossible goals as you will always be disappointed.
- The mind always tries to achieve what is expected of it.
  Think of failing and you are more likely to fail.
  Think of nothing and your mind will be bored.
  Think of succeeding, and you are more likely to do so.
- Everyday do something you want to do, as opposed to something that you have to do.
- If you tend to do everything yourself, ask for help or give responsibility to others sometimes.
- Consider yourself as well as others. You have needs too.
- Share your feelings with other people.
- Do not expect to be perfect in the future. Perfection is impossible.
- Do not be rushed all day with no time to think or feel. Aim to be quiet with your thoughts for part of each day.
- Live in the present more than in the past or in the future.
- Compliment others when they deserve it and be happy with them.
- Responsibility is good as long as there is neither too much nor too little.
- Continual whining makes problems bigger, not smaller.
- Hope is an excellent bridge.
- With others it is important to be co-operative, but that does not mean that you always give in. Say 'no' sometimes and be a good listener.
- If no one can help or understand you, you are not communicating.
- Other people have problems too.
- Think about what you want to do with your life. It would be a pity to get to the end and wish you had lived it entirely differently.
- You have a problem? Consider it, read about it, think about it, talk about it. Try going round it, over it, or under it. If all else fails, go right through it, but do not spend your whole life looking for it.
- Worry is an unhealthy, destructive, mental habit and a waste of time.
- Never take anxiety or worry to bed with you. They will snore all night.
- Thoughts about situations or people you do not like or can't change need to be thrown out. Thinking about them wastes your life and no one else's.
- Believe in yourself and rebuild your immune system with a well-balanced diet of healthy thoughts; then peace, happiness, love, health and humour will smile with you.

14

ACT AGAINST AIDS

H IV stands for human immunodeficiency virus and is the virus which causes AIDS. Individuals may be infected with the virus ie be HIV positive but not develop the disease Acquired Immune Deficiency Syndrome for a number of years. Why do some people who are HIV-positive remain fit and healthy for many years while others go on to develop AIDS comparatively quickly? At present nobody knows for sure but after a decade of concentrating on drug therapy alone, doctors are beginning to realise that they may have to look further afield for some of the answers. Research has finally begun to focus on the patients themselves and the state of their natural immunity and resistance to disease. Scientists are considering a range of co-factors, such as diet and lifestyle, which may be vital in determining whether a person infected with HIV will develop full blown AIDS.

It is becoming clear that one very important co-factor is impaired nutritional status. Some researchers have suggested that malnutrition could influence both susceptibility to HIV infection and progression of the disease. One study concluded that nutritional status is strongly associated with survival. It also found malnutrition to be widespread and severe at the time of diagnosis. Other research suggests that depleted nutrient levels result from the actions of the virus and malnutrition is a well documented consequence of AIDS. Weight loss, body cell mass depletion, decreased skinfold thickness and mid-arm muscle circumference, decreased iron-binding capacity and selenium deficiency are frequently reported in the AIDS population. The extent of body cell mass depletion has been found to correlate with death.

The cause of impaired nutritional status could be increased and un-met nutrition needs, decreased nutrient intake or malabsorption. Research is increasingly suggesting that a good nutritional status does have a beneficial effect on response to treatment and could help people with AIDS to maintain their quality of life.

The importance of early nutritional intervention in HIV infection has been recognised by doctors in the United States where most of the research has been carried out. Several studies have suggested the importance of aggressive nutritional intervention and a report commissioned by the American Food and Drug Administration strongly recommended nutritional screening of people who are HIV+ along with early nutritional intervention, counselling and education about diet.

A study based on data from the San Francisco Men's Health Study suggested that a number of nutrients might reduce the progression to AIDS in people with HIV. A total of 296 men, all healthy and HIV-positive, were enrolled in the study which lasted six years. During that period 36% of them progressed to AIDS. With some statistical adjustments, the research seemed to demonstrate that the risk of AIDS decreased as consumption increased for all 10 micronutrients (vitamin A, (carotene, retinol), vitamins C and E, folic acid, riboflavin, thiamine, niacin, iron and zinc). This relationship was statistically significant for iron, vitamin E and riboflavin and approached significance for vitamin C, thiamine and niacin. A higher intake of all 10 micronutrients was associated with higher CD4 counts and was significantly so for six of them. Daily multivitamin use was associated with a 33% reduced risk of developing AIDS.

However, because of difficulties interpreting the data, the researchers were cautious in their conclusions, saying only that "the possibility that higher nutrient intakes may delay the development of AIDS cannot be ruled out".

Dr Richard Beach from the University of Miami School of Medicine says that patients frequently arrive very depleted in overall nutritional status. He believes it is important to start early nutritional intervention. "Our studies show people are frequently deficient in zinc, selenium, copper, B6 and B12 even while remaining asymptomatic" he says. "In patients with AIDS, nearly every specific nutrient is deficient." He found that 20 to 40% of the asymptomatic patients he studied had abnormally low plasma levels of riboflavin, vitamins A, B6, C, E, zinc and copper. 25% of them had a vitamin B12 deficiency and were found to have low scores when tested for information processing speed and visual/spatial ability. Upon correction of B12 levels, performance in these areas normalised.

Other studies have also found evidence of B12 deficiency. Researchers at the University of Rochester School of Medicine found 20% of patients referred for neurological evaluation had abnormal B12 metabolism associated with peripheral neuropathy and myelopathy. They tended to be older people, in the later stages of HIV infection. Most of them had AIDS. The researchers concluded that B12 deficiency may be a frequent and treatable cause of neurological dysfunction in patients with HIV and recommended routine evaluation of B12 levels in patients where a distal sensory motor neuropathy develops. They suggested the likelihood of this deficiency increases with the progression of immunosuppression and recommended replacement therapy which has few associated toxic side effects and may significantly improve neurological function.

Neurological manifestations of B12 deficiency can include dementia with the usual symptoms of slowed mental reaction, confusion, memory defects and depression all of which frequently appear in AIDS-related dementia. Symptoms of peripheral neuropathy include the types of leg and foot pains experienced by many AIDS sufferers.

A decrease in B12 associated with bone marrow toxicity has been reported with the use of AZT and one researcher has suggested that substantial quantities of B12 may reduce the anaemia which can be caused by AZT.

Dr Beech believes the lack of another B vitamin (pyridoxine, B6) can be directly correlated to decreased immune system activity and he suggests the deficiency is directly related to the anxiety and depression often experienced in early HIV infection.

There is evidence that antioxidant substances may be beneficial in cases of HIV infection. Vitamin C is a powerful immune-stimulating and virus-inhibiting nutrient which strengthens the body's resistance to disease. Researchers from the Linus Pauling Institute in California have shown vitamin C's ability to suppress the HIV virus in laboratory cultures of infected cells. They found that with continuous exposure to ascorbate, in concentrations not harmful to cells, the growth of HIV in cultured human lymphocytes could be reduced. A later study confirmed that the continuous presence of ascorbate was necessary because when it was removed, the virus began to replicate again.

Leading researcher, Dr Raxit Jariwalla suggests that in healthy humans, based on pharmaco-kinetic data, a dose of 12 grams administered orally is needed to obtain the minimum blood levels for anti-viral effect.

Dr Robert Cathcart is an American physician who has been treating immunosuppressed patients for some years. He says that when a person is ill, the body pool of vitamin C is rapidly depleted and processes that depend on adequate tissue levels of C, including some needed for immune response, are put at risk of malfunctioning. He is convinced that AIDS can cause this depletion. "The sicker the patient gets, the more ascorbate is destroyed in the disease process," he maintains.

Cathcart is a long time advocate of large doses of vitamin C, which he says can suppress the symptoms and reduce the incidence of secondary infections. His preliminary clinical evidence is based on experience with over 250 HIV-positive patients and it suggests that depletion of CD4 T-cells is slowed, stopped or sometimes reversed for several years when doses close to tolerance are maintained. The dosage seems to be critical because it is only when it reaches 80-90% of bowel tolerance that any effect is observed on acute symptoms. Dosage is increased until the patient experiences mild diarrhoea and then reduced slightly. This point is known as bowel tolerance.

The amount of vitamin C which can be tolerated orally by a patient, without producing diarrhoea, increases somewhat proportionately to the toxicity of the disease. However, Cathcart cautions that prolonged administration of large amounts of any nutrient should only be done in consultation with a specialist to avoid induced deficiencies in other nutrients.

The deleterious effects of vitamin C megadoses which have been reported include gastrointestinal disturbances, a rise in serum cholesterol and destruction of vitamin B12. There have also been reports that large doses can cause kidney stones but the most recent literature indicates there is little risk of this.

N-acetyl-cysteine (NAC), a sulphur-containing derivative of the amino acid cysteine, is another powerful antioxidant under investigation. Many HIV-infected individuals have low levels of glutathione in their body and NAC has been shown to raise these levels.

Glutathione, a tri-peptide made up of the three amino acids cysteine, glutamic acid and glycine, acts as an antioxidant protecting the cells against toxic compounds including heavy metals and excess oxygen. It enhances immune function and is important in the initiation and progression of lymphocyte activation. It is also critical for the function of natural killer cells and research has suggested that a deficiency may contribute to the immune dysfunction of HIV and influence the progression of AIDS. One study carried out on monkeys, suggests that reduced intracellular glutathione is a direct and early consequence of retroviral infection.

In addition to its glutathione inducing properties, NAC has been shown to detoxify harmful chemicals and protect the body against heavy metals such as mercury, lead and cadmium, along with herbicides and other environmental pollutants.

It also appears to have other benefits. A study at Boston University School of Medicine, found that NAC could enhance T cell colony formation *in vitro* and concluded that it might be able to enhance T-cell numbers in patients with AIDS or ARC. Other research has shown its ability to protect against some of the damage caused by radiation which may be particularly beneficial to patients undergoing radiotherapy for conditions such as Kaposi's sarcoma.

Perhaps even more significantly, NAC was also found to have anti-viral properties and in further studies at the Linus Pauling Institute, Dr Jariwalla and his research associate discovered that by adding vitamin C to NAC a synergistic effect was created that caused an eight-fold increase in anti-HIV activity. The combination of NAC and vitamin C was twice as effective as vitamin C alone.

In the United States, PWA's have been using NAC since 1988. Anecdotal reports are generally good although not particularly dramatic. People often report feeling better and having more energy, an effect likely to occur within several days of starting the treatment. The San Francisco-based newsletter Aids Treatment News suggests that NAC may be especially useful for certain people with AIDS-related wasting which is not due to obvious problems such as inadequate food intake or gastrointestinal disease.

In the absence of clinical trials there is no recommended dosage as yet. According to researcher and author Dr Richard Passwater, early indicators from laboratory studies suggest that clinically effective amounts may be in the range of four grams of NAC daily. He cautions that ingestion of 150mg per kilogram of body weight or more may produce adverse effects such as cellular necrosis. "Appropriate clinical studies need to be conducted to determine efficacy and safety," he says.

Digestion of fats is frequently another problem area for PWA's and the immune system can be affected by the type of fats consumed. Researchers from the Royal Free Hospital in London and the University if Miami in Florida as well as doctors in Rome, have all reported depleted levels of essential fatty acids (EFA's) in patients with AIDS and they conclude that viral disturbance of the metabolism of essential fatty acids occurs with HIV infection and may be a cause of some of the observed symptoms.

In a study carried out at the Muhimbili Medical Centre in Dar Es Salaam, 12 patients with AIDS diagnosed on the basis of evidence of HIV infection from a blood test, severe weight loss, and at least two other major symptoms were selected. They were given capsules containing EFA's derived from a mixture of evening primrose oil and fish oil. At the end of 12 weeks, the patients had put on weight and experienced considerable improvement in their symptoms with a reduction in fatigue and diarrhoea and an improvement in skin rashes. Moreover there was a significant improvement in the CD4 lymphocyte count from 59 to 261/mm. None of the patients experienced any adverse effects with this treatment.

Approximately 20 months after starting the EFA study, five of the twelve patients remained alive and relatively well, which, according to Dr David Horrobin, one of the researchers, is an unusual survival rate for this region, where patients usually delay seeing their doctor for as long as possible. One report suggests the survival rate for people in this region with AIDS, once they go to the doctor, is only 63.5% after one week and only 7.5% at the end of three months.

At the University of Dar Es Salaam, a larger placebo-controlled study using EFA's has recently been completed. This has shown good results which will be published next year in 1997.

Thanks to Peter Sofroniou for authoring this chapter.

15

WINNING THE COLD WAR

re you a favourite host for the cold virus? Do you stock up on boxes of tissues, and make Tunes a part of your daily diet when winter comes along? If so, now is the time to strengthen your defences and make yourself virus-proof. There are basically two methods of defence. The first is to prevent infection in the first place. The second is to minimise the effect of infection once it occurs.

Viruses are not technically 'alive' as they cannot reproduce. They can only multiply if they get inside your cells and get these invaded cells to make more viral particles. In order to keep viruses out you need to have sufficient vitamin A in your body and enough calcium and magnesium to make those cell walls strong enough to resist the virus.

At the onset of winter, the external temperature gets colder and the body becomes less able to use its supply of vitamin A. This starts a vicious circle with vitamin A becoming more and more in demand. This is probably one of the reasons why zinc is helpful when you've got a cold because it allows vitamin A, stored in the liver, to be used.

The secret of any battle is to be well prepared. Start now by making sure that you have adequate nutrients to keep your immune system at the ready. Your multivitamin supplement should contain at least 7,500 iu of vitamin A and at least 1,000mg of vitamin C as well as a good B complex (one which contains choline, pantothenate and folic acid). Your multimineral should contain zinc but not copper and at least half as much magnesium as calcium. If you're a person who often suffers from infections you may need to experiment with a maintenance dose of up to 20,000 ius of beta-carotene, which is a non-toxic form of vitamin A, and an additional 3 grams of vitamin C.

Is your early warning system on alert?

As with any attack the element of surprise gives a distinct advantage and unfortunately it is usually in the favour of the attacking virus. How do you know that they have arrived? The first cause for suspicion is if you've been in the company of someone with a cold. Symptoms usually start two or three days after exposure. You also have your own 'early warning system' that tells you when you have unwelcome guests. The warning signs are a sensation in the throat or nose on waking, a thick head or a hint of a headache, heavy muscles, feeling slightly tired even before you get up or feeling hot, cold or shaky. If you feel these symptoms don't hesitate to reach for the vitamin C. Even if it turns out to be a false alarm you can only benefit.

Why enough vitamin C is essential

So many proper research trials have shown that large amounts of vitamin C lessens the frequency, shortens the duration and lessens the symptoms of a cold. A recent review of sixteen such studies showed that, on average, 34 per cent less days of illness are experienced by those who supplement vitamin C. So why do so many doctors still sneeze at vitamin C for colds? There are an equal number of papers that show no effect. However, a close look at these papers shows two common fundamental flaws. In some studies laboratory bred viruses are squirted up the poor subject's nose. These viruses are so virulent and numerous that it's little wonder vitamin C shows no effect. It's a bit like testing a boxer's mouthguard by hitting him in the face with a sledgehammer! The more frequent blunder is a failure to administer enough vitamin C. The best results have been achieved using between 400mg and 1,000mg per hour. According to Dr.Linus Pauling "The amount of protection increases with the amount of ingested vitamin C taken at the immediate onset of a cold." In fact, the amount needed depends very much on the person. A good policy is to take 3g immediately and 2g every four hours until symptoms subside, which should be within 24 hours. Before going to bed take a further 3g. Although you can lessen the dose on subsequent days it is definitely wise to keep supplementing more than usual vitamin C for two days after symptoms have stopped. Stopping vitamin C suddenly can result in a return of symptoms. You may experience loose bowels on these large amounts, but that is all. There is no harm from taking large amounts of vitamin C for a few days.

In the long-term supplementing 1 to 3g of vitamin C every day helps to keep your immune system strong. It is probably best to supplement this with other nutrients needed to maintain a healthy immune system. One such supplement, Immunade, which provides vitamin A, E, zinc, selenium, calcium, magnesium and molybdenum as well as 1g of vitamin C, was tested in a double-blind trial at ION involving 37 people. After twelve weeks 81 per cent of those taking Immunade considered themselves less susceptible to colds, compared to 44 per cent on a placebo tablet. The incidence of cold symptoms and the duration of symptoms were also considerably reduced in the Immunade group.

Seven ways to stop a cold dead in its tracks

1 Take 3 grams of vitamin C immediately and then two grams every four hours (or three times a day). Alternatively, mix 6 grams of vitamin C powder in fruit juice diluted with water and drink throughout the day. Some people prefer to use calcium ascorbate, a less acidic form of vitamin C.

2 Also supplement other immune boosting nutrients especially vitamins A and E, selenium, and zinc.

3 Eat lightly, preferably relying mainly on fruits and vegetables, including foods rich in vitamins A and C, for example carrots, beetroot, green peppers and citrus fruit.

4 Avoid mucus forming and fatty foods, i.e. meat, eggs and milk produce. These make your lymph limp - and lymphatic fluid is the main transport system for immune cells which carry invading viruses to lymph nodes for further punishment.

5 Avoid all alcohol, cigarettes, tea and coffee. Drink plenty of water and herb teas.

6 Take it easy. Do everything slowly and avoid stressful situations. Get some rest and plenty of sleep.

7 Once you think you've won wait at least 24 hours then cut the vitamins down to 1 gram of vitamin C three times a day, and one immune boosting vitamin and mineral supplement in the morning. Once you have been well for three days go back to your normal supplement programme.

Part 4

IMMUNITY AND NUTRITION

16

FIGHTING FOOD

When you think about it, Nature has the perfect system cracked. It provides foods in seasonal rotation so that we do not become sensitive to them. It provides foods packed with immune power boosters in late summer and autumn when we need them to build up for the winter ahead, when the cold and flu bugs traditionally play 'hunt the human'. All vegetable matter can be recycled either by passing through animals or by rotting, so releasing vital minerals back into the soil (unless you put your vegetable rubbish in plastic bags in the dustbin, of course).

Man knows best, or thinks he does

• Seasonal food is now available all year round, either we preserve it or import it.

• Man is obsessed with storing food. It can now be stored for so long that there are few, if any vitamins left in it.

• Nutrients are often taken out of food by various processing methods in order to increase shelf life, after all no self respecting bug would want to eat nutrient deficient food. Given the choice, bugs will inhabit the nutrient packed whole foods first, causing them to spoil and leave the processed, nutrient deficient stuff for those intellectually superior humans.

• We spray various pesticides on our food to stop other things from eating our precious stores, regardless of the fact that they are poisons and will have some effect on us too. Other sprays which are not poisonous in themselves, destroy vitamins eg. methyl bromide and some of the chlorinated hydrocarbons completely destroy all of the vitamin B5 or inositol, respectively.

• Soil and crops are covered with so many chemicals that wise worms wriggle long distances to pop into the organic farm next door.

• Despite all of the added chemicals, some that we do need are not replenished, either because they are too expensive or because they do not effect the look of and yield of the crop, eg. selenium and zinc.

• The worth of a pound of human flesh has increased in money terms with our increased intake of lead, mercury, aluminium, cadmium and nickel, but was it worth the deleterious effects it has had on human health?

The food we eat affects our thoughts, behaviour, mood and temper, our ability to exercise, relax and sleep. It alters our hormones, skin, blood, organs, bones, muscle and fat, in short, it provides the building blocks of our life and we determine whether we build ourselves a short term, shaky shack or a strong and durable castle. Very roughly speaking, we change our bodies almost entirely throughout a seven year period. Whatever we have now can be improved on with a little (or a lot of) maintenance during that time. Alternatively we can allow ourselves to crumble and fall into disuse and disrepair. The choice and responsibility are ours. Refined, processed, nutrient deficient foods give us inferior building blocks. We may be able to build a large house, especially if we eat a lot of them, but will it last? How strong is it? Does everything inside and out work properly? Will it take the test of time or will it only take a little wolf to huff and puff and expose our unhealthy bacon?

We use food as materials for making the weapons of our immune army and the quality of our defence when we go to war rather depends on whether we have the materials to build water pistols or nuclear weapons.

There are two main types of people who are particularly at risk. Together they make up quite a sizable portion of the world's population - they are the needy and the greedy. These people all suffer from malnutrition. They either do not have enough food to eat, and insufficient variety to provide all of the nutrients necessary, or they eat far too much of the nutrient deficient foods. Foods themselves need nutrients in order for the body to be able to use them properly. Sugar and alcohol for example both need B vitamins and yet these are refined out of them. Both conditions contribute to a suppressed immune system.

A general recipe for a sound immune system

Assuming you are not on any special diet for medical reasons, these guidelines could be applied daily for a lifetime.

• Of the total calorific intake 60% is best taken in the form of carbohydrate, mainly wholefoods and comprising grains other than our national addiction, wheat, along with lots of fruit and vegetables.

• Not much more than around 20% should come from fat, but one has to ensure that this includes the essential fatty acids, especially linoleic (eg. sunflower or safflower oils) and EPA (eg. seafood) or another omega 3 oil perhaps flax seed oil or borage oil if you are vegetarian or don't like fish.

• The remaining 20% should provide all of the amino acids to make up complete protein.

• Mix with care and cook only when necessary.

• Eat only when hungry.

• Avoid the use of seasoning such as artificial chemicals or salt.

• Sprinkle liberally with immune boosting herbs:

H for humour - many people forget it at the back of the cupboard.

E for enthusiasm - we all have it but often lose it.

E for exercise - we all need it but often neglect it.

E for encouragement - we should all give it and receive it.

R for right thinking - a positive attitude to problems.

R for relaxation - to balance stress.

B for balance - the key to health but difficult to achieve all of the time.

S of sociability - people need people.

S for supplements - to make up for the nutrients missing in your diet or to counteract any toxic ones put in.

17

THE MAGIC AND MENACE
OF MINERALS

When we take in minerals we take in compounds, eg. common salt is made up of two elements, which gives the compound or mineral-sodium chloride. The following list gives the elements which are either required by the immune system or hinder it:

Calcium

Calcium has so many functions in the immune system including:
• Needed by all phagocytic cells in order to attach to and ingest foreign material.
• Cytotoxic T cells need calcium in order to make the enzymes which kill.
• Complement proteins cannot join together without calcium and so would remain inactive.
• Calcium is needed to destroy viruses.
• Calcium is needed for fever production, this in turn means that macrophages can move faster and produce destructive enzymes more efficiently.
• Also many viruses cannot replicate at an elevated temperature.
Good food sources are:
• Fish, especially those with bones you can eat.
• Grains and bread.
• Beans, soya beans, peanuts, seeds.
• Dairy produce, milk, cheese, yoghurt etc.
There are a lot of calcium robbers eg. coffee, chocolate, toxic minerals, high fat diets, oxalic acid (rhubarb), bran, high protein diets, medical conditions associated with poor absorption.

Magnesium

- Needed for complement fixation.
- Needed for cell mediated immunity.
- Needed for maintaining the thymus.
- Needed to maintain antibody levels.
- A deficiency could cause a rise in histamine levels and hence increase allergic reactions.
- Needs to be in balance with calcium and phosphorus. Those on a fast food and soft drink diet get a very heavy dose of phosphorus. Magnesium is, conversely, very low in the typical British diet.
- Those who take extra calcium to guard against osteoporosis and joint problems, should also take extra magnesium or they may get an increase in arthritic pain and unnecessary calcification.

Good food sources are:

- Nuts and seeds (sesame seeds have about the best calcium/magnesium balance).
- Green vegetables.
- Corn.
- Some fruits, apple, fig and citrus.
- Hard water. (Not, of course, if you use a filter or water softener.)

Iron

The right amount of iron boosts overall resistance to infection, but too much is actually bad for the immune system. Iron found in food has low toxicity so iron rich foods are preferable to supplements and some poor supplements contain the form of iron which cannot be utilised by the body anyway, rather like sucking a rusty nail - also not recommended. Vitamin C enhances absorption of iron from food.

Iron is essential for antibody production. Iron is needed for production of enzymes produced by macrophages and PMN's. Myeloperoxidase, an iron containing enzyme, is used to make white blood cells. Iron is needed for the detoxification of some drugs and bacterial toxins.

Bacteria, however, cannot usually reproduce without iron, so avoid iron containing supplements or iron-rich foods when suffering from a bacterial infection. Leucocytes (our white blood cells) produce an iron-binding protein when we have a bacterial infection, to tie up iron, so there is no sense in giving it more and overworking the system at this time.

Iron deficiency is relatively common in children and pregnant women, probably because pregnant women need that little bit more for foetal development and children are notorious for disliking green vegetables and offal which are very rich food sources! Grains, cereal and bread are reasonable sources, if not refined, as are egg yolks and peaches.

Selenium

Our daily requirement of this is very small, around 50 micrograms which, put in perspective, is about a millionth of our daily protein needs. It is, however, needed and deficiency is associated with cancer. British soil has very low levels of it, it is not added in fertilisers and we have one of the highest cancer rates. Natural food sources are best such as nuts, seeds, wholegrain cereals and seafoods. Fruit and vegetables would be if grown in selenium rich soils.

Don't however, take regular, high dose supplements (above 200mcg) as more is definitely not better. Too much can be toxic. It is used in antibody production and is a very good antioxidant, working well with vitamin C. Research on animals has shown that there is no antibody production at all when animals are deprived of vitamin E and selenium. It has been suggested that these two, given at the time of vaccination, could increase antibody production and hence the effectiveness of the vaccine. White blood cells lose their efficiency in recognising invaders without it.

Zinc

Deficiency causes atrophy of the thymus, (the master gland that vets all of our T cells), possibly due to the fact that it is needed for normal release of vitamin A from the liver. (Vitamin A and zinc work synergistically.)

It is needed to produce enzymes that help eliminate routinely produced cancer cells, not for the large amounts once cancer is established. It is found in over 200 of the body's known enzymes. The hormone thymulin, which is necessary for T cell maturation, is also zinc dependent.

Zinc is high in, but lost with, seminal fluid, so men with high sexual activity need more zinc. Deficiency shows up as white spots in the nails and a decline in the senses of taste and smell. It is quite a common deficiency as water pipes these days are often made from copper and this is taken into the water, especially in soft water areas. Whilst not a problem in itself in that the body needs some copper too, we do need a rough balance of zinc/copper intake, just as we need a calcium/magnesium/phosphorus balance.

Main food sources are meat, especially organ meats, shellfish, eggs, leafy green vegetables, (although Britain again has quite low levels of zinc in the soil and it is not added with fertilisers). Seeds are probably the best source, especially pumpkin seeds.

Monster minerals

Not all elements are required by the body, in fact some can interfere with its normal processes and so are termed antinutrients. Antinutrients always have a detrimental effect on the immune system, either directly or because they interfere with the uptake of nutritional ones. Calcium, iron, magnesium, selenium and zinc are often pushed out by the toxic bullies like aluminium, arsenic, cadmium, lead, mercury, fluorine and nickel.

Although nickel, arsenic and fluorine are used in minute amounts our problem is always excess. Smoking and heavy margarine consumption contribute to nickel overload whilst chocolate, beer, shellfish and meat may contain arsenic if the raw material from which they are made or fed was sprayed with arsenic based insecticide. Fluoride is often, unfortunately, put into the water supply. It's in most toothpastes in this country, although it has been banned in other countries, and is also used as an insecticide and rat poison. We are getting far too much of it.

The body has no choice but to accept aluminium, cadmium, lead and mercury, although they can only do harm. A good analogy is that they are like keys which fit into the locks of some of our enzyme systems but unlike the nutritional key which fits the lock and opens the door, the anti-nutrient merely fills the keyhole so that the proper key cannot be put in. It will not open the door! We cannot totally avoid antinutrients but we need to try to keep them to a minimum.

18

VITAL VITAMINS

To be able to adjust diet and supplements, it is necessary to know what the various nutrients do for the immune system. It is now well known that deficiency or excess of many micronutrients cause the body to malfunction. Outright deficiency diseases like scurvy (vitamin C), are relatively rare in this country today. We are now more likely to suffer from marginal deficiencies of several vitamins.

Vitamin A

This is known as the growth vitamin because it is necessary for the production of the growth hormone, which in turn is responsible, not only for growth, but for maintaining an active thymus and hence a strong immune system. T cells will obviously be depleted if growth hormone is in short supply as the thymus will have shrunk, it will be less active and so will be less efficient at maturing T cells. B cells are also adversely affected.

Vitamin A is a powerful antiviral vitamin, mainly because its inclusion in cell walls makes them stronger and more resistant to viral attack. It is particularly important for strong linings in areas of special risk from infection, such as the respiratory system, the gut and the genito-urinary tract.

Body secretions like sweat, tears and saliva, as well as the immune system's cells, all contain lysozyme and need vitamin A for the production of this protective antibacterial enzyme. Along with vitamin C, vitamin A is probably deficient in individuals who regularly suffer from conjunctivitis.

Vitamin A's precursor, beta-carotene, is being researched because of its possible role in preventing and treating cancer and for use after major surgery.

Vitamin A and beta-carotene must combine with bile salts in the gut in order to pass into the bloodstream. If someone is on a very low fat diet, bile does not reach the intestine and over 90 per cent of the vitamin A may be lost in the faeces. Furthermore, vitamin E intake is crucial to prevent destruction of vitamin A before it can be utilised or stored.

Foods rich in vitamin A
• Eggs.
• Milk fat, butter, cream.
• Fish oils and oily fish.
• Liver, kidney.

Foods rich in beta-carotene
• All green vegetables, such as spinach, cabbage, endive, lettuce, kale, broccoli, legumes.
• Cashew nuts and beans.
• Carrots, swedes, corn, pumpkin, sweet potato and peppers.
• Cherries, cantaloupe melon, water melon, peach and papayas.

When you need more
• If suffering from an infection, especially a viral infection.
• If suffering from cystic fibrosis.
• If suffering from atherosclerosis.
• If diabetic, you would need preformed vitamin A (retinol). More care is needed not to over - supplement the preformed variety.
• If the system is coping with the intake of mineral oil, perhaps as a laxative. (It is not a good idea to consume mineral oil for any reason.)
• If deficient in protein, as vitamin A is needed for its synthesis.
• If the diet is rich in protein, as protein requires vitamin A for its utilisation.
• If vegetables, fruit and fish are not a major part of the diet.
• If suffering from skin conditions (psoriasis, acne etc.)
• If you smoke; the mucus lining of the respiratory tract is damaged by smoke and lots of vitamin A is used up in repairs.
• If you live in an heavily polluted area - exhaust fumes destroy vitamin A.
• If bladder stones are a problem.
• If you are under a lot of stress, which will increase adrenal activity and decrease the thymus. Vitamin A is needed to reverse this.

• During winter the body is less able to utilise vitamin A in cold conditions. Perhaps this is why the polar bear stores so much, (polar bear liver is toxic to humans because it is so high in preformed vitamin A). It is protective against hypothermia for elderly people; it is important that they take extra during the winter months.

• Males who are impotent may suffer from vitamin A deficiency.

• Alcoholics need extra vitamin A.

• If you have been exposed to a carcinogen, the waiting period (preneoplasia), which may be up to 20 years from exposure to the manifestation of cancer, is probably the time when vitamin A exerts most of its protective effect and prevents malignancy.

Symptoms of deficiency
• Poor growth in children.
• Poor night vision.
• Mouth ulcers.
• Skin complaints, from dandruff to acne.
• Genito-urinary infections or vaginitis, especially in the elderly.
• Susceptibility to viral infections in general.
• Decline in sense of taste, smell and hearing.
• Lack of tears and extreme sensitivity to light.
• Improper tooth and bone formation.

Supplements
When supplements of vitamin A are needed, they are best taken in the form of beta-carotene as this form is not toxic and is only made into vitamin A as required. Diabetics need performed vitamin A or cod liver oil as they cannot convert beta-carotene into vitamin A. Supplements need to be taken with a little fat and vitamin E to be effective.

B complex vitamins
Bacteria need B vitamins, so do not bother to take B supplements during a bacterial infection. They are also important for every cell of the body, and that includes those of the immune system, where they build better resistance. They are particularly important for mucus membranes. Folic acid and pyridoxine (B6) probably have the most effect on the immune function.

Folic acid is essential for pregnant mothers and for the development of mature organs in the fetus. It has been found that the thymus is larger and the immune system stronger if the mother has had a good supply of folic acid, choline, B12 and methionine. Folic acid is also necessary for all cell division, and hence is of particular importance, not only for the infant, but also whenever there is a need for healing.

A B6 deficiency causes a decrease in the activity of the phagocytic cells so that we cannot clean up inside as effectively as we should. Remember, phagocytes get rid of old, dead cells and any other unwanted matter.

Choline used to be included as a B vitamin. It changes into dimethyl-glycine in the body. This substance increases lymphocyte production three or four times in comparison with a deficient animal. It is also a natural detoxification supplement.

Food sources

Major food sources are liver, yeast, blackstrap molasses, and whole grains, especially, wheatgerm and rice bran.
• **B1:** Offal, pork, beef, whole grains, nuts, legumes and sunflower seeds.
• **B2:** Liver, milk, meat, leafy green vegetables and sunflower seeds.
• **B3:** Organ meats, meat, peanuts, legumes, milk, eggs, tuna and sunflower seeds.
• **Folic acid:** Dark green vegetables, organ meat, beans, whole grains, salmon, tuna, dates and milk.
• **B6:** Molasses, offal, whole grains, green vegetables, peas and prunes.
• **B12:** Milk and dairy produce, fish, offal and eggs.
• **B5:** Yeast, green vegetables (especially broccoli), cashew nuts, milk, eggs, mushrooms, nuts, salmon and seeds.
• **Choline:** fish, eggs, offal, yeast and peanuts.
• **Biotin:** Organ meats, molasses and milk.
• **Inositol:** Organ meats, molasses, whole grains, nuts.
• **Pantothenic acid:** Yeast, whole grains, meat, organ meats, nuts, peas, beans, dates and cauliflower.

When you need more

• Women suffering from premenstrual tension (PMT) often need more.
• Pregnancy or the use of oral contraceptives increases the need for folic acid and B6.

- Conclusion of a course of antibiotics.
- Pantothenic acid (B5) is often deficient in allergic bottle fed babies.
- Hypoglycemics need extra pantothenic acid.
- Heavy refined-sugar eaters need more B complex; in fact heavy eaters in general need a lot of B vitamins, especially if consuming refined foods.
- Anyone taking cortisone is probably deficient in B5.
- Really overweight people who fast or who drastically cut down on food without adding B vitamins, especially B5, can get symptoms of arthritis or gout. B vitamins should always be added when slimming as they are required for the proper breakdown and utilisation of body fat.
- Alcoholics are B deficient.
- The adrenal glands can produce sex hormone-like substances; these are invaluable to a woman after the menopause, and help to prevent osteoporosis, as long as they are not exhausted by tea and coffee drinking combined with a deficiency of pantothenic acid.
- Tannin in tea is an anti-B1 agent; heavy tea drinkers need more B vitamins.
- Radiotherapy sickness is sometimes alleviated using B6 with a low dose B complex under medical supervision.
- Children on soya-milk diets are often B deficient, B2 in particular. It firsts manifests itself as red, watery eyes.
- People with high cholesterol levels require extra niacin.
- Those who suffer with indigestion daily are often B deficient and cannot make the hydrochloric acid necessary for digestion in the stomach.

Symptoms of deficiency
The B vitamins are used by just about every cell in the body, and they are used in a lot of the body's chemistry, so their deficiency symptoms are very varied, although almost always there are mental effects such as depression, anxiety, difficulty with concentration and moodiness. There is often also an energy problem, because B vitamins are needed to make energy from food; without them, lack of energy or tiredness are inevitable.

A host of other symptoms may also be evident, like headaches, premenstrual tension (PMT), bad breath, dandruff, eczema, water retention, weight problems, sensitivity to light and so on.

Probably one of the most reliable physical guides to B vitamin inadequacies is the mouth, and in particular the tongue; cracked sore lips and mouth corners; tongue enlargement or decrease in the size of the tongue itself or of the taste of the buds on it; deep fissures or, alternatively, a very smooth sore tongue; coatings, smell or off-colour tongues are telling you that you are B deficient. The obvious deficiency in the mouth will be extended to other areas of digestion. Stomach acid production and enzymes will be insufficient and the chances are there will be excessive gas and indigestion.

Gut bugs also need B vitamins to do their housework in the intestines; without their contribution, this area will not be kept as clean as it could be and, after a long period of deficiency, could well become a slum area.

Supplements

To supplement the diet it is better to take a B complex, including a good balance of them all. Taking one or two only increases the need for the others, and having a poor balance can create as many problems as it may solve; vitamin B2 and B6 intake in particular must be about even.

A B50 complex is a usual supplement, containing 50 mg of each of the main B family. B100's may be necessary for a period if there is severe deficiency or if a course of antibiotics has just been finished - medication such as antibiotics, sulphonamides and others destroy B vitamins.

Sometimes a single B vitamin is supplemented for a short time to restore a balance. It should always be taken with a low dose B complex or with plenty of B-rich food.

Vitamin C

Vitamin C has so many functions in the immune system including:

• Vitamin C is an antiviral. Many viruses such as flu and the common cold do not necessarily enter the bloodstream. They spread from cell to cell in the mucus secretions on the respiratory tract membranes. Consequently there is a very little antibody stimulation. Defence falls to cell-mediated T lymphocytes to do their job and reduce the symptoms.

• Prostaglandin E production in the blood platelets is boosted by vitamin C, and this in turn increases the T-lymphocyte production. The greater the number and effectiveness of any army, the better the chance of victory.

• Vitamin C is needed for a special kind of cell division called phytohaemagglutinin- induced blastogenesis, which results in a rapid increase of lymphocytes, both B-cell and T-cell types. The flu virus actually works by depressing this type of cell division. Vitamin C supplementation switches it back on again.

• Interferon production is greater with sufficient vitamin C. It is produced by the infected cell and causes a further protein to be produced by itself and neighbouring cells which blocks the synthesis of essential viral proteins. As viruses cannot replicate themselves, but need the host cell to do it for them, it stands to reason that the greater the production of interferon, the less the cells will make the virus.

• Vitamin C can be bacteriostatic or bactericidal, depending on the bug. Most bacteria require B vitamins for their life processes, but not vitamin C - the latter can seriously hinder bacterial growth and multiplication. It can even kill some bacteria under the right conditions.

• C3 complement production is improved with vitamin C and this in turn triggers B lymphocytes to manufacture more antibodies, especially IgA, IgG and IgM.

• It stimulates non-lysozyme antibacterial factor (NLAF) found in tears. This is of obvious importance for people who often suffer from eye infections.

• Vitamin C enables those leucocytes responsible for engulfing foreign particles to carry out their function. Leucocytes can only perform phagocytosis if they contain at least 20 micrograms of vitamin C per 100 million cells.

• Vitamin C detoxifies, partially at least, many bacterial toxins, depending on the bug involved. It is often the toxin which causes all the unpleasant symptoms.

• Apart from stimulating natural antibacterial factors in the body, vitamin C will actually improve the performance of antibiotics.

• Mononuclear phagocytes, a special type of white blood cell, use vitamin C with hydrogen peroxide and some minerals, especially zinc compounds, to kill the invaders that they have captured. Research shows that zinc has a role to play in the prevention of colds, especially if sucked slowly with vitamin C.

• Vitamin C also helps sore eyes and runny nose, as it is a natural antihistamine.

• Vitamin C obviously has a great effect on the immune system, but dose is important - it will vary from individual to individual. If a cold or any other form of infection catches you, increase your supply until it is over, then gradually decrease your dosage again.

Most animals have an enzyme called L-gluconolactone oxidase which allows them to make vitamin C. Man, along with guinea pigs, the Indian fruit-eating bat and the red vented bulbul bird, do not. All these rely on vitamin C in their diet and all die of scurvy without it. Man can make very small amounts from folic acid, because folic acid is converted in the body to its biologically active form, tetrahydrofolic acid and ascorbic acid; unfortunately folic acid is also commonly found to be deficient and only supplied in micro amounts, so we get very little vitamin C this way.

Irwin Stone, an eminent biochemist, postulated that during evolution man lost his ability to make ascorbic acid in sufficient quantities due to a mutation in the gene that makes the particular liver enzyme L-gluconolactone oxidase. He suggested that the mutation did not pose any threat at the time, because man was a great fruit eater and had plenty of vitamin C in the diet. Now, however, it is a different matter. Storage and processing deplete our food of vitamin C, and we eat less fresh fruit than our ancestors did. Other animals, like the gorilla, living in the wild, consume about 4.5 grams of vitamin C daily in fresh food. Other mammals too, saturate blood and tissue with vitamin C and step up their production when they are ill or under stress. It is possible that infectious diseases, cardiovascular disorders, collagen diseases, cancer and premature aging are among the many ills which could be prevented if we still had the ability to regulate our vitamin C levels.

Whilst many studies confirm benefits with supplemental vitamin C, others do not, probably due to the fact that the dosage has to be sufficient for any given person at any given time - it is very difficult to judge the correct amount.

Bowel tolerance is a useful general indication of vitamin C requirements. A normal, young, healthy adult will tolerate 1 to 4g of vitamin C before getting diarrhoea. If the patient has flu, this tolerance may go up to 4 to 8g, while if he has cancer or AIDS, he may require 20 to 30g a day. It all depends on the individual, which makes research a little more difficult.

Age is another major factor; our absorption of vitamin C goes down considerably with age, though in old animals its production is not that much different to that in young animals. Older people need more vitamin C spread out in small amounts over the day.

Needless to say, a lot of work has been done on guinea pigs, as they most closely resemble us as far as vitamin C utilisation is concerned. For example in very low vitamin C diets, cholesterol formation in their adrenal glands went up 600 per cent and their ability to heal wounds was poor.

It is known that during phagocytosis oxygen is used up, hydrogen peroxide is produced and used to destroy the germ which has been captured and the hexose monophosphate shunt (the chemical process whereby the cell gets more energy from glucose) is speeded up. Researchers have found that this activity is low in normal, healthy white blood cells, but is speeded up, by up to six times the norm, when they are infected. The speed was greater when vitamin C was added. In those with scurvy or those who are vitamin C deficient, the white blood cells engulf bacteria but cannot digest them or destroy them. Vitamin C reverses this cellular indigestion.

Food sources
Most fresh fruits are very good sources of vitamin C, especially oranges, kiwi and melon, as long as they have not been kept in storage for too long. Most vegetables are also good sources, especially greens, broccoli, tomatoes and peppers.

When you need more
• During the winter, intake may be stepped up for protection against colds and flu; and it should be stepped up a lot if exposed to these viruses or if initial symptoms are felt.
• Those who both smoke and drink alcohol need more vitamin C as it is known to help detoxify acetaldehyde. Smokers on average have 25 per cent less vitamin C in the blood than similar non-smokers who are on the same diet. Heavy drinkers also need extra vitamin C and zinc as both are necessary for the production of alcohol dehydrogenase, the liver enzyme which detoxifies alcohol.
• Diabetics cannot transport vitamin C across cell membranes very well, and side effects such as poor wound healing can be helped by supplements of vitamin C.

• Aspirin depletes the body's vitamin C reserves, so these should be replenished by those on aspirin therapy.

• The need for vitamin C in the diet increases with age.

• High cholesterol levels may be lowered with sufficient vitamin C. Research shows that a normal guinea pig converts 40 per cent more cholesterol to a safer form than does one which is deficient in vitamin C. It also tends to have less atherosclerosis than deficient ones.

• Most medical drugs destroy vitamin C in the body, although many of them are first detoxified by it. The destructive effect, however, may go on for some weeks after the drug is discontinued. Drugs are sometimes necessary and life saving, so it is probably wise to increase vitamin C intake if you have to take them.

Symptoms of deficiency
• Easy bruising
• Bleeding or receding gums.
• Slow healing.
• Frequent infections.

Supplementation
Supplements are best taken with bioflavins, or food containing them. Vitamin C or ascorbic acid powder is the cheapest and purest form in which to buy this, as it does not have the fillers and binders which would be needed to make tablets. If ascorbic acid is not well tolerated by the stomach (it sometimes causes heartburn), the more gentle calcium ascorbate can be used; this is not acidic, and can be mixed with water, or orange juice in the same way.

Many people like to take vitamin C daily but it can also be used as a 'medicine' by increasing the dosage if illness does threaten. Always remember to take it with a lot of fluid and to decrease the intake gradually when an infection has passed, rather than to stop suddenly.

Vitamin D
Vitamin D, when taken in excess suppresses the immune system. People who suffer from conditions that already suppress their immune system are generally advised to avoid supplementation. However, it must be remembered that vitamin D is essential for healthy bones, and hence for

normal movement. Indirectly the immune system suffers if bones are unhealthy and you can not move freely, because it is muscular contraction and movement which pushes lymph around the body.

Japanese studies show that a daily supplement of around 500iu of the natural form of vitamin D3 may help to reverse the disturbed helper/suppressor T cell ratio which occurs in chronic fatigue syndrome.

I am a firm believer in sunshine for many reasons, and this is one. When the sun's ultraviolet light hits the skin, it changes the form of cholesterol in the skin into cholecalciferol, which is the natural form of vitamin D (also known as D3). Other D's, namely D2, D4, D5 and D6, are synthetic versions and have greater side effects than the natural D3 (which is also found in fish oil).

Our skin colour determines the amount of ultraviolet light (UV) we let through and the amount of vitamin D made. Black skin only allows 3 to 36 % of the UV through, whilst white skin allows 52 to 72 % to be absorbed. As white skin tans, the amount of UV allowed through is reduced, so offering protection from damage which could cause skin cancer, and regulating the amount of vitamin D made. In general, we make less vitamin D in winter, because we have less exposure to sunlight; supplemental fish oil during the winter months is therefore quite a good idea for children and the elderly in particular, because bone needs calcium, magnesium and vitamin D for growth and repair. Many of the degenerative bone problems could be avoided with the right diet, exercise and exposure to sunshine.

We also need to have the immune system suppressed sometimes. After an infection has passed, for example, we need to be able to turn off the immune system; this requires suppressors. It is the right balance that we are aiming for, and the right amount of vitamin D is needed to play its part.

Food sources
- Cod liver or halibut liver oils.
- Oily fish.
- Egg yolk.
- Milk.

When you need more
• If already suffering from osteoporosis or degeneration of the spine.
• If you spend a lot of time indoors or are bedridden.

Supplements
Natural supplements like fish oil are the best.
Vitamin D is fat soluble and so is stored in the body. It is possible to take too much, so sunlight and fish should be used where ever possible and only supplemented when really necessary.

Vitamin E
Unfortunately, these days we seem to be obsessed by increasing the shelf life of foods so that they keep longer than the people who eat them. Vitamin E is an essential nutrient, but is often removed if the food is to be kept for a long time; although a natural antioxidant, it goes off faster than artificial ones which are used to replace it.

Vitamin E is necessary for a normal antibody response. As an antioxidant in our fat layers, it neutralises free radicals and works with other nutrients to improve our resistance to infection. It is very effective in protecting us from air pollution, particularly that due to exhausts, air purifiers or deodorisers which generate ozone.

Food sources
• Whole grains - rice, wheat, wheatgerm, oats.
• Cold-pressed oils - sunflower, safflower.
• Green leafy vegetables.
• Eggs and liver.

Supplements
Supplements should be built up gradually, 100 iu at a time, to a maximum of 1,000 iu. Although good for heart complaints, people suffering from these should be especially wary to include this vitamin only gradually and with professional advice. Vitamin E may reduce the need for drugs like anticoagulants.

19

ACE ANTIOXIDANTS

During the last decade more and more research has confirmed that many of the 20th century's most common diseases are associated with deficiency of antioxidant nutrients, and helped by their supplementation. A new medical model is emerging, that considers the presence of any one of these diseases as a sign of probable antioxidant deficiency, in the same way that scurvy is a sign of vitamin C deficiency. In the future we may be tested for blood levels of antioxidant nutrients, alongside blood sugar, cholesterol and blood pressure. Capable of predicting your biological age, and expected lifespan, your antioxidant nutrient status may prove to be your most vital statistic.

Medical literature is replete with information which suggests that a common denominator in the aging process and the diseases associated with aging is 'oxidative damage'. This has put the spotlight on the use of antioxidants, nutrients that help protect the body from this damage, in the prevention and treatment of disease. So far, over a hundred antioxidant nutrients have been discovered and hundreds, if not thousands of research papers have extolled their benefits. The main players are vitamins A, C and E, plus beta-carotene, the precursor of vitamin A found in fruits and vegetables. Their presence in your diet, and levels in your blood may prove the best marker yet of your power to prevent death and disease.

What is an antioxidant ?

Oxygen is the basis of all plant and animal life. It is our most important nutrient, needed by every cell every second of every day. Without it we cannot release the energy in food which drives all body processes. Oxygen is chemically reactive and highly dangerous. In normal biochemical reactions oxygen can become unstable and capable of 'oxidising' neighbouring molecules. This can lead to cellular damage, triggering cancer, inflammation, arterial damage and ageing. Known as

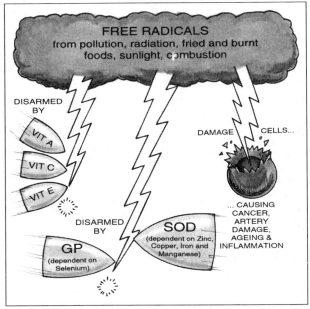

How antioxidants disarm free radicals

'free oxidising radicals' this equivalent of 'nuclear waste' must be disarmed to remove the danger. Free radicals are made in all combustion processes including smoking, exhaust fumes, radiation, fried or barbecued food and normal body processes.Chemicals capable of disarming free radicals are called 'antioxidants'. Some are known essential nutrients, like vitamins A & beta-carotene, C and E. Others are not essential as such, like bioflavonoids, anthocyanidins, pycnogenol and over 100 other recently identified protectors found in common foods.

The balance between your intake of antioxidants and exposure to free radicals may literally be the balance between life and death. You can tip the scales in your favour by simple changes to diet and antioxidant supplementation.

The big jigsaw put together from available research seems to show that antioxidants play an important role in the progression of many major diseases. Overleaf are examples of some research findings:

Antioxidant Related Diseases

Alzheimers	Cancer
Cataracts	Cardiovascular disease
Diabetes	Hypertension
Infertility	Macular degeneration
Measles	Mental illness
Periodontal disease	Respiratory tract infections
Rheumatoid arthritis	

Alzheimers
Elderly people with Alzheimers disease have lower blood vitamin A levels, half the vitamin E levels and less than half the beta-carotene levels of elderly people who don't.

Cancer
People with lung cancer have much lower blood vitamin A levels. Those with low dietary intake of vitamin A have double the risk of lung cancer than those with the highest vitamin A intake. Similarly, a high intake of beta-carotene from raw fruits and vegetables reduce the risk of lung cancer in nonsmoking men and women. Supplementing beta-carotene (30mg per day) resulted in 71% of patients with oral precancer (leukoplakia) improving, while patients given 200,000iu of vitamin A a day resulted in 57% of patients having complete remission.

Cataracts
People with low blood vitamin C levels have 11 times the risk of developing cataracts compared to those with high blood vitamin C levels. Similarly, those with low vitamin E blood levels had almost double the risk. People consuming 400ius of E a day have half the risk.

Heart disease and high blood pressure
The higher your vitamin A levels (63 to 83µg%) and vitamin C levels (0.7 to 0.9µg%) in the blood, the lower your risk. Also, in the case of vitamin C, the lower your blood pressure. Supplementing 1,000mg of vitamin C also reduces blood pressure. One study of nurses showed that those who consumed 15 to 20mg per day of beta carotene had 40% lower risk of

stroke and 22% lower risk of a heart attack compared to those consuming 6mg per day. Those with high dietary intakes of beta-carotene halved their risk of death from cardiovascular disease. Supplementing 500mg of vitamin E reduces risk of a heart attack by 75%.

Infertility

Supplementing 20 infertile men with 1g of vitamin C produced conception in all their couples within 2 months. Not so for those on placebo.

Macular degeneration

People with macular (eye lens) degeneration have lower blood vitamin E and vitamin C levels. Those with high beta carotene levels have half the risk of developing it.

Mental Illness

The manic/depressive state of 24 people was vastly improved within hours of supplementing 3 grams of vitamin C.

Immunity and infections

Supplementing 800 ius of vitamin E daily, increases blood levels and immune response; 180mg of beta carotene daily, increases immunity and T-cell count. Supplementing vitamin A (450µg per day) reduced the incidence of respiratory tract infections on pre-school children.

Rheumatoid arthritis

Supplementing 1,200mg of vitamin E reduced pain and stiffness in patients with rheumatoid arthritis.

Many disease conditions are associated with specific nutrient deficiency. Supplementing the related nutrient improves the condition but will only do so if a deficiency was all or part of the problem in the first place. Infertility in men, for example, has many different possible causes some of which are physical and not related to nutrition at all. These will obviously not be helped by increased nutrient intake.

Many other diseases not listed here, including colds, diabetes, HIV infection, measles, periodontal disease and chronic fatigue syndrome are also associated with antioxidant deficiency. *The above information, compiled, with credit and thanks to Dr Emanuel Cheraskin, is a summary of 40 research papers, first published in the Journal of Orthomolecular Medicine 10:2, 1995, p89-96. This paper is available from ION for £1. Please send an SAE.*

Supplements - How much?

VITAMIN A - The Suggested Optimal Nutrient Allowance per day for vitamin A and beta-carotene is 800 to 1,000mcg RE (retinol equivalent) for children and 800-2,000mcg RE for adults. ION recommends supplementing between 2,000mcg (6,600iu) and 3,000mcg (10,000iu) per day of retinol and the same again for beta-carotene.

VITAMIN C - The Suggested Optimal Nutrient Allowance per day is 150mg for children and 400 to 1,000mg for adults. ION recommends supplementing between 1,000 and 3,000mg per day.

VITAMIN E - The Suggested Optimal Nutrient Allowance per day is 70mg for children and 90 - 800mg for adults. ION recommends supplementing between 265mg (400 iu) and 670mg (1,000 iu) per day.

Antioxidants - The Best Foods

The best all-round antioxidant foods have the highest •••• rating.
Foods are listed in order of their ••• rating.

FOOD _Rich source of_	A	C	E
Sweet potato	•••	•	•••
Carrot	•••	•••	
Watercress	•••	•••	
Peas	•	••	••
Broccoli	••	•••	
Cauliflower	•	•••	
Lemons	•	•••	
Mangoes	••	••	
Meat	••		••
Melon	••	••	
Peppers	•	•••	
Pumpkin	••	••	
Strawberries	•	•••	
Tomato	••	••	
Cabbage	•••		
Kiwi fruit	•	••	
Oranges, grapefruit	•	••	
Seeds & nuts			•••
Tuna, mackerel, salmon			•••
Wheatgerm			•••

Your Personal ANTIOXIDANT Profile

Test your Power of Prevention

SYMPTOM ANALYSIS

____ Do you frequently suffer from infections (coughs, colds)?

____ Do you find it hard to shift an infection?

____ Do you have a recurrent infection (cystitis, thrush, earaches etc.)?

____ Do you bruise easily?

____ Have you ever suffered from any of the conditions listed overleaf?

____ Have your parents collectively suffered from two or more of these conditions?

____ Do you easily get exhausted on physical exertion?

____ Does your skin take a long time to heal?

____ Do you suffer from acne, dry skin or excessive wrinkles for your age?

____ Are you overweight?

Add up your score out of 10. 1 for each 'yes'.

LIFESTYLE ANALYSIS

____ Have you smoked for more than 5 years of your life, less than 5 years ago?

____ Do you smoke now?

____ Do you smoke more than 10 cigarettes a day?

____ Do you spend time most days in a smoky atmosphere?

____ Do you have an alcoholic drink each day?

____ Do you live in a polluted city, or by a busy road?

____ Do you spend more than two hours in traffic each day?

____ Are you quite often exposed to strong sunlight?

____ Do you consider yourself unfit?

____ Do you exercise excessively and get easily 'burnt out'?

Add up your score out of 10. 1 for each 'yes'.

DIET ANALYSIS

_____ Do you eat fried food most days?

_____ Do you eat less than one serving of fresh fruit and raw vegetables each day?

_____ Do you eat less than two pieces of fresh fruit a day?

_____ Do you rarely eat nuts, seeds or wholegrains each day?

_____ Do you eat smoked, barbecued food or grilled cheese on your food?

_____ Do you supplement less than 500mg of vitamin C each day?

_____ Do you supplement less than 100iu of vitamin E each day?

_____ Do you supplement less than 10,000iu of vitamin A or beta-carotene each day?

Add up your score out of 8. 1 for each 'yes'.

Your TOTAL SCORE

0-10

This is an IDEAL score, indicating that your health, diet and lifestyle is consistent with a high level of antioxidant protection. Keep up the good work!

11-15

This is a REASONABLE score, although you can increase your power of prevention by converting 'yes' answers into 'no'.

16-20

This is a POOR score, indicating much room for improvement. See a nutritionist to upgrade your diet and lifestyle for increased antioxidant protection.

20 +

This is a BAD score, putting you in the high risk group for rapid ageing. See a nutritionist and ask for an Antioxidant Profile blood test. You'll need to make changes to your diet and lifestyle, plus supplement antioxidants to reverse or slow down the ageing process.

20

THE FATS OF LIFE

A lot of work has and is being done on the role of vitamins, minerals and essential fatty acids in preventing, alleviating or curing medical conditions. Research has been able to show just where and how these food factors are utilised in the body and hence we have a clearer picture of when and under what conditions we need to increase or decrease their intake. Fats have been studied a lot recently due to their probable role in causing heart and circulatory diseases.

What is fat?

The term used for all of the fat like substances is lipid. Lipids are divided into fats, (solid at room temperature) and oils (liquid at room temperature). They are very important in body structure, as they are part of the membrane that surrounds every single cell in the body. With the right sort of lipids the cell membranes are strong, without it they are weak and more prone to attack. It is also an important component of brain and nervous tissue. Probably the best known phospholipid is phosphatidylcholine and an enzyme which attacks this is the active ingredient of the venoms of many poisonous snakes and insects.

In Britain we eat, on average, 125 grams of fat a day and we are being advised to reduce this to 100 grams. or 25-30% of our calorie intake. Not only that but we have to watch the types of fat we eat. There are saturated fats, which are mainly of animal origin. Then there are monounsaturated fats, the obvious example being olive oil which is mainly the monounsaturated, oleic acid. They only have one double bond and are not associated with any risk of heart disease. Finally there are polyunsaturated fats which have more than one double bond and are associated with a decreased risk of heart disease, although an increased risk of cancer, if used a lot heated (and reused). This is due to the production of free radicals at high temperatures and free radicals are considered to be cancer inducing.

How much fat is in your food?

	Fat content%		Fat content%
Bacon, sausages	50	Beef, lamb, pork	20
Brazil, pecan, hazelnut	over 60*	Butter	80
Chocolate	40	Cottage cheese	4
Coconut	35	Chicken, tuna	10
Crisps	40	Eggs (whole)	12
Hake, haddock	1	Hard cheese	30
Lard	100	Mackerel & herring	25
Margarine	80	Mayonnaise	80
Milk (whole)	3.7	Oats	5
Pastry	50-33	Sesame seed, sunflower seed	45*
Thick cream	40		

mainly polyunsaturated

Fats are about twice as high in calories as proteins or carbohydrates and make up 38 to 40 per cent of our total calorie intake. This is really much too high. People in third world countries consume far less than 20 per cent, but they are at the other extreme. The ideal fat content of our diet is probably somewhere between 25 and 30 per cent of our calorie intake. Most people neither have the time nor the inclination to count the calories they eat, work out the fat content and turn it into percentages. So it is easier to use a rough guide. Those foods that are less than 20% fat (by weight, not calories) can be used as part of the everyday diet without too much concern. Those that are above this level need a lot more thought as to balance and quantity; for example, crisps, chocolate bars and sausages should not be staples of our diet, although, unfortunately, they are becoming so for many of our children. These foods are all high in calories, high in fat, high in salt or sugar and low in nutrients - just the ingredients for a short, unhealthy life. There is no reason, however, why they cannot be enjoyed occasionally.

Why eat fat at all?

Even if we eat no fat, we will make it from excess carbohydrates and proteins; for example, the latter can be converted into fat if we eat more than we need for growth, repair and topping up our amino acid pool.

The body cannot, however, make the essential fatty acids, and these have to be supplied in the diet to maintain health and normal body weight.

The body needs fat - for padding and shape, and to protect bones, nerves, blood vessels and internal organs. It is also needed as insulation, in order to maintain a constant body temperature and for immediate as well as stored energy. However its use as a reserve food, i.e. as a long-term energy reserve, is rarely needed in this country.

In order for fat to be both built up and broken down properly, other nutrients are required, in particular linoleic acid (itself an essential fat), the B group of vitamins (especially choline and inositol) and magnesium. Without sufficient of these extra substances, it may be very difficult either to put weight on (if you are too thin), to take weight off (if you are too fat) or to metabolise and store fat properly.

In digestion, we break fats down into their building blocks and then use these blocks to build up what we need again. Our efficiency at breaking down and building up fat is crucial to our health and shape, and is nutrient dependent.

Types of fat we eat

Saturated fats
Saturated fat is solid at room temperature, and is mainly of animal origin. Coconut and palm fat are the two exceptions; they are cheap and often used in food processing. Coconut fat is almost entirely saturated fat. All saturated fats are good for business, because they are consistent - cakes or biscuits will always taste the same, packet after packet - and have a long shelf life. Chip-shop vegetable fat is often palm or mixed fat.

Mono-unsaturated fats
People of the Mediterranean area eat about 30% of their total calories as fat, but their diet is low in saturated fat. They use a lot of olive oil which is a mono-unsaturated fat. Mono-unsaturated fats are good to cook with as there is only one double bond which can be broken to give undesirable free radicals. It does not appear to be linked with any risk of heart disease or cancer.

Polyunsaturated fats
Heart disease is a major killer and has been linked to our saturated fat consumption. To try to get the right balance, we have been encouraged

to eat more polyunsaturated fat, which is needed by the body to transport such things as fat-soluble vitamins.

To further complicate the issue, there are essential fatty acids which are needed by the body but cannot be made or converted from existing fats; they have to be consumed. These are essential for good immune function, blood clotting, nerve impulses, brain function, intestinal fitness, regulation of fat metabolism, transport of cholesterol and the integrity of the cell membrane.

The three important ones are:

• Linoleic acid, belonging to the omega 6 group of fatty acids. Foods rich in this are seeds and their natural oils, nuts, wheat and oatgerm. Chicken and pork have more linoleic acid than lamb, beef or deer because bacteria in the rumens of the latter animals convert it into saturated fat.

• Arachidonic acid, also belongs to the omega 6 group of fatty acids but is not as desirable as the above because we tend to eat too much of it. It's a question of trying to restore the balance. It's found in meat and dairy produce, which are consumed a lot in this country.

• Alpha-linolenic acid, belonging to the omega 3 group of fatty acids, is found in green vegetables, flax seed oil, blackcurrant seed oil, soy oil and phytoplankton. As the latter is the staple diet of many fish, these in turn are rich in the Omega 3's.

EFA's and the prostaglandins

All of the essential fatty acids give rise to groups of chemicals known as the prostaglandins. These prostaglandins (PG's) have various effects on the body:

• The one series of prostaglandins (PG1) is involved in the regulation of the T-suppressor lymphocytes and in a decrease in the stickiness, or the ability to clot, of the blood. They therefore decrease the risk of heart disease.

• The two series of prostaglandins (PG2), which includes a subgroup called the leukotrienes, are known to increase inflammation and blood clotting. Furthermore, the leukotrienes are involved in asthma and other allergic conditions.

• The three series of prostaglandins (PG3), reduce the clotting tendency of blood.

These three groups of prostaglandins are derived from the three essential fatty acids:

- The PG1 series is derived from linoleic acid.
- The PG2 series is derived from arachidonic acid.
- The PG3 series is derived from alpha-linolenic acid.

It is therefore important to balance the intake of the various essential fatty acids in order to ensure a beneficial balance of the prostaglandins in the body, such that blood clotting and the inflammation response are available at a suitable level when needed, but are not available in excess so that they cannot cause blood clots and inflammation for no reason. For example, a diet rich in a mammalian meat tends to produce an overload of the PG2 series and the leukotrienes, which in turn tends to increase the risk of heart disease. A deficiency of the PG1 series also tends to be present in people with autoimmune diseases like rheumatoid arthritis, as well as in those with multiple sclerosis; this is thought to be due to the effect these prostaglandins have on the T-suppressor cells. Interestingly, aspirin is often used to treat heart disease and rheumatoid arthritis, reducing inflammation by preventing the formation of PG2 prostaglandins from arachidonic acid.

Essential fatty acids

Most people are deficient in both Omega 6 and Omega 3 fats. In addition, a high intake of saturated fats and damaged polyunsaturated fats, known as 'trans' fats, stops the body making good use of the little essential fats the average person eats in a day.

The 'Omega 6' fat family

The grandmother of the Omega-6 fat family is linoleic acid. Linoleic acid is converted by the body into gamma-linolenic acid (GLA), provided you've got enough vitamin B6, biotin, zinc and magnesium to drive the enzyme that makes the conversion. Evening primrose oil and borage oil are the richest known sources of GLA and, by supplementing these direct you need take in less overall oil to get an optimal intake of Omega 6 fats. The ideal intake is probably around 150mg of GLA a day, which is equivalent to 1,500mg of evening primrose oil, or 750mg of high-potency borage oil - a capsule a day.

GLA then gets converted into DGLA and from there into

Omega 6 Deficiency Signs

Do you have high blood pressure?
Do you suffer from PMS or breast pain?
Do you suffer from eczema or dry skin?
Do you suffer from dry eyes?
Do you have an inflammatory health problem, like arthritis?
Do you have difficulty losing weight?
Do you have a blood sugar problem or diabetes?
Do you have multiple sclerosis?
Do you drink alcohol every day?
Do you have any mental health problems?
Do you suffer from excessive thirst?

How do you score? Five or more 'yes' answers indicates that you may be deficient in Omega 6 fats. Check your diet carefully for the foods listed below.

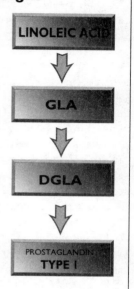

'prostaglandins' which are extremely active hormone-like substances in the body. The particular kind of prostaglandins made from these Omega 6 oils are called 'Series 1 prostaglandins'. These keep the blood thin, relax blood vessels, lower blood pressure, help to maintain water balance in the body, decrease inflammation and pain, improve nerve and immune function and are essential for insulin to work properly and maintain good blood sugar balance. This is the short-list. As every year passes more and more health-promoting functions are being found. Prostaglandins themselves cannot be supplemented as they are very short-lived. Instead we rely on a good intake of Omega 6 fats from which the body can make the prostaglandins we need.

This family of fats comes almost exclusively from seeds and their oils. The best seed oils are hemp, pumpkin, sunflower, safflower, sesame, corn, walnut, soybean and wheatgerm oil. About half of the fats in these oils come from the Omega 6 family, mainly as linoleic acid. An optimal intake would be about 1 to 2 tablespoons a day, or 2 to 3 tablespoons of ground seeds.

The 'Omega 3' fat family

The modern day diet is likely to be more deficient in Omega 3 fats than Omega 6 fats simply because the grandmother of the Omega 3 family, alpha-linolenic acid, and her metabolically active grandchildren, EPA (eicosapentaenoic acid) and DHA (docosahexaenoic acid), from which Prostaglandin Series 3 are made, are more unsaturated and more prone to damage in cooking and food processing. As these fats get converted in the body to more 'active' substances, they become more unsaturated and generally the word used for them gets longer (e.g. oleic acid - one degree of unsaturation; linoleic - 2 degrees of unsaturation; linolenic - 3 degrees of unsaturation; eicosapentaenoic - 5 degrees of unsaturation etc.). You can see this increasing complexity as we move up the food chain. For example, plankton, the staple food of small fish, is rich in alpha-linolenic acid. Carnivorous fish, like mackerel or herring, eat the small fish who have converted some of their alpha-linolenic acid to more complex fats. The carnivorous fish continue the conversion. Seals eat them and have the highest EPA and DHA concentration, then Eskimos eat the seals and benefit from the ready-made meal of EPA and DHA from which they can easily make the series 3 prostaglandins.

These prostaglandins essential for proper brain function, affect vision, learning ability, co-ordination and mood. They reduce the stickiness of blood, as well as controlling blood cholesterol and fat levels, improving immune function, metabolism, reducing inflammation and maintaining water balance.

The best seed oils for Omega 3 fats are flax (also known as linseed), hemp and pumpkin. In much the same way as evening primrose oil bypasses the first 'conversion' stage of linoleic acid, eating carnivorous fish or their oils bypasses the first two conversion stages of alpha-linolenic acid, to provide EPA and DHA. This is why fish eaters like the Japanese have three times the Omega-3 fats in their body fat than the average Westerner. Vegans, who eat more seeds and nuts, have twice the Omega 3 fat level in their body fat than the average Westerner.

Essential balance

While borage oil or evening primrose oil may be the best source of Omega 6 and fish oil the best source of Omega 3, that doesn't make them the best allrounders. The ideal source of essential fats should have high levels of both. Differing views exist about the ideal ratio. Estimated intakes of our hunter-gatherer ancestors suggest that we need equal amounts. The ratio found in blood even of high fish eaters is about 5 times as much Omega 6, suggesting that it is either relatively more important, or that all cultures have a relatively greater deficiency of Omega 3 fats. Some researchers advise that we may need to take in twice as much Omega-6 as Omega 3 to match our relative need. Either or these ratios is a long way off the average diet, which is deficient in both.

The best allrounder is hemp seed oil from the marijuana plant. Hemp has been grown for many years. The fibre is used to make rope, the seeds can be used to make hemp butter and the leaves are a good fertiliser. It is, however, illegal to grow in many parts of the world. The seeds and fibre are legal, neither of which will make you high, and can therefore be

Omega 3 Deficiency Signs

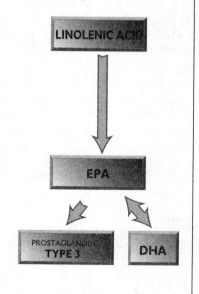

Do you have **dry skin**?
Do you have any **inflammatory** health problems?
Do you suffer from **water retention**?
Do you get **tingling** in the arms or legs?
Do you have **high blood pressure** or **high triglycerides**?
Are you prone to **infections**?
Are you finding it harder to **lose weight**?
Has your **memory and learning ability** declined?
Do you suffer from a **lack of co-ordination** or **impaired vision**?
If a child, are you small for your age or **growing slowly**?

How do you score? Five or more 'yes' answers indicates that you may be deficient in Omega 3 fats. Check your diet carefully for the foods listed below.

imported into the UK. Hemp seed oil is 19% alpha-linolenic acid (Omega 3), 57% linoleic acid and 2% GLA (both Omega 6). It is the only common seed oil that meets all known essential fatty acid needs. Hemp seed oil is not easily available in the UK.

Another way of meeting the needs for both Omega 3 and Omega 6 fats is to combine seeds. Sunflower and sesame are good sources of Omega 3, pumpkin provides reasonable quantities of both, and flax seed is richest in Omega 3, being approximately 50% Omega 3 and 10% Omega 6. Put 1 measure each of sesame, sunflower and pumpkin seeds and 2 measures of flax seeds in a sealed jar and keep it in the fridge, away from light, heat and oxygen. Simply adding 2 tablespoons of these seeds ground to your breakfast each morning guarantees a good daily intake of essential fatty acids. Alternatively, add 1 and make up the difference with a salad dressing, nuts or seeds later in the day.

Of these seeds the most unsaturated is flax seed, so it's most prone to damage. For this reason it's important to buy fresh seeds that have been properly stored, minimising heat, light and oxygen exposure. A small number of companies offer seed oils that are processed in such a way as to protect the oils from oxidation. We recommend you only buy oils that are extracted from organic seeds, cold-pressed to minimise heat, and stored in a light-proof container, preferably flushed with nitrogen to exclude any oxygen. In this case a good daily balance of essential fatty acids could be obtained by 1 tablespoon of flax seed oil or a high potency capsule of EPA/DHA **plus** 2 tablespoons of ground seeds (e.g sesame, sunflower, pumpkin) or a high potency primrose or borage oil capsule.

Each of the following provides your daily need for these essential fatty acids. Individual needs do vary so this is only a rough guideline.

OMEGA 3	OMEGA 6
2.5% to 5% of total calories	5% of total calories
8 to 17 grams a day	17 grams a day
Flax seed Oil: 1 tablespoon	Evening primrose oil: 1,000mg
Flax seeds: 2 tablespoons	Borage oil: 500mg
EPA/DHA: 1,000mg	Sunflower seeds: 1 tablespoon
Pumpkin seeds: 4 tablespoons	Pumpkin seeds: 2 tablespoons
	Sesame seeds: 1.5 tablespoons

21

PROTEINS AND CARBOHYDRATES

I f you answer yes to a lot of the questions in the box overleaf, you could be protein deficient. Surprisingly, there are quite a few people who are deficient in protein, even in a country like ours which appears to have ample food. Water retention in pregnancy may well signal protein deficiency, as insufficient albumin may cause a problem with picking up waste water from tissues. People on unbalanced slimming diets, vegans or vegetarians who have just decided to adopt that lifestyle but have not bothered to learn about amino acid combining, fast food addicts, people who live alone and children are most at risk.

Children and young people need a lot of protein for growth; however, many chose a low-nutrient fast-food diet; Some become vegetarian when their parents are not, and so tend to be given the same meals, but without the meat. Yet others are put on restrictive diets by parents.

What are proteins?

Protein is the basic constituent of all living cells. Three-quarters of the dry weight of most body cells is protein. Proteins make up hormones, enzymes, neurotransmitters and antibodies. The name comes from proteus, a mythological figure who, like protein, could change his form. If we eat cow protein or bean protein, we break it down into its constituent amino acids and then make it up again into the protein we require. The amino acids themselves perform essential functions. Some control depression, memory, sleep, moods, energy levels, relaxation, tension, the immune response and so on.

An adult builds tissue and changes his body roughly every seven years. This is of course an over-simplification in that the brain cells cannot be replaced and bone collagen takes more like 30 years to replace, but at the other end of the scale we get a new skin every three or four

Protein Deficiency

- Do you find it difficult to hold yourself up straight when sitting or standing?
- Do you have rounded shoulders, a sunken chest or flat feet?
- Do your hair and nails grow slowly?
- Do you have difficulty concentrating?
- Do you get short periods of depression, anxiety and irritability?
- Is your memory slipping?
- Do you have difficulty sleeping?
- Do you get frequent infections?
- Do you get wandering aches and pains?
- Do you feel that you look older than you are?
- Do you constantly feel hungry?
- Does your mood change frequently?
- Do you have weight problems?
- Do you get indigestion?
- Do you have very low blood pressure?
- Do you suffer from constipation?
- Do you suffer from water retention?

weeks and two new gut linings every week. Every second, normal bone marrow makes about two and a half million new red blood cells. Every second, we create around 200,000 new immune cells, and thousands of antibody molecules. Our spares and repairs department need an awful lot of amino acid building blocks.

The amino acids

There are eight essential amino acids which are vital to life. Our friendly gut bugs make very small amounts for us all of the time, and without this background level we would suffer from severe mood swings. Antibiotics often cause mood problems as a result of loss of gut bug production.

The essential amino acids mostly lacking in plants are methionine, tryptophan and lysine. The first, methionine, is essential for a pregnant woman because a baby's thymus and immune function is dependent on it. Soya beans and legumes are deficient in methionine. All cereals are deficient in lysine.

All living things require certain amino acids more than others. Babies and children need histidine and arginine in addition to the eight essentials, and pre-term babies require cysteine and taurine. Cancer cells have their favourite diet; melanomas, for example, can be starved by withholding their chosen addiction, phenylalinine and tyrosine. The central nervous system is regulated to a large degree by amino acids, and amino acid therapy is being used increasingly in the treatment of many psychiatric disorders. In their role as neurotransmitter, proteins take on the job of vital communicators.

Amino acids are also the 'written codes' on substances, allowing the body's immune system to recognise them as self or to destroy them as rubbish or potential enemies. Antibodies, too, are protein, and lymphocytes have a high requirement for amino acids for their production and function. The amino acids which stimulate the immune system most are alanine, aspartic acid, cysteine, glycine, lysine, methionine and threonine. Those used for detoxification include glycine, methionine, cysteine, glutamine, taurine and tyrosine.

Patients with liver disease, gallbladder problems, diabetes, hypoglycaemia, aggressive behaviour, or addictions may all be helped using various combinations of amino acids. It should be remembered

Amino Acid Therapy

- Alanine, carnitine, leucine, isoleucine and valine are commonly used for muscle building.
- Methionine, taurine, carnitine, arginine and glycine are used to bring down cholesterol and triglyceride levels.
- Phenylalanine, tryptophan, arginine, carnitine and gamma-amino-butyric acid (GABA) are used as appetite suppressants.
- Methionine, tryptophan and d-phenylalanine are used to control pain.
- Tryptophan, GABA and glycine relieve insomnia.
- Even serious diseases like Parkinson's disease can be helped by such amino acids as tryptophan, tyrosine, L-dopa, methionine, GABA and threonine.
- Stamina can be increased using carnitine and dimethyl glycine.

however, that this is using amino acids as drugs and they should be taken under medical direction. I am a firm believer in real food. If it is eaten whole, already packaged with the nutrients it needs for its utilisation, many of these imbalances would not occur in the first place. It is very easy to create an imbalance in the body's amino acid pool, but not so easy to sort it out. For this reason I include here only a few of the amino acids, in general terms, as they apply to the immune system.

Methionine

Scientists tried to imitate what they thought was earth's primitive atmosphere. The atmosphere contained carbon, hydrogen, nitrogen, oxygen and sulphur in combination, and a spark in it formed methionine. This, plus the fact that methionine is the essential methyl donor to bacteria, leads one to conclude that it is our oldest amino acid, essential and very useful. Sunflower seeds and cottage cheese are probably the richest natural sources, and egg is also good, but potatoes are deficient.

Methionine relieves pain and is a component of various endorphins (these are chemicals involved in feelings of happiness and well being). It is very important in metabolism and enzyme systems and essential for the foetal immune system. It is also very important for the immune systems of children; I note this, as some children are put on soya bean diets (no milk or meat), and soya bean is very deficient in methionine - in fact, it is probably the limiting factor in many soya-based infant formulae. Methionine deficiency might not be noticed until the baby grows into a more sickly child.

Experiments on monkeys show that a deficiency of methionine causes atherosclerosis. Children and pregnant mothers in particular need foods sufficient in methionine.

Cysteine and glutathione

Cysteine is very important for the immune system, mainly because it is synthesised into glutathione in the body. Its level is quite high in a normal thymus.

Millions of years before life on earth, our atmosphere was probably toxic. When life did begin, it had to develop a protection. It is essential to our immune systems today, because, yet again, we have a lot of toxic substances in the air, both gases and heavy metals. Provided there is sufficient cysteine present, the body increases its levels of glutathione when it is trying to cope with excess lead, mercury, cadmium or arsenic; it is also thought to help with detoxification of exhaust fumes and pesticides within the body.

Glutathione is an anti-oxidant and helps protect us (and plants) against toxic forms of oxygen. It is, in fact, such a primitive and universal anti-oxidant that it has even been considered as an additive to dying lakes to restore life there. It is poorly absorbed, because there used to be sufficient of it, but a calorie-sufficient, though nutrient-deficient, modern diet may not be providing enough.

• Glutathione is necessary for macrophages, in order to make the chemicals they need to kill invaders, for lymphocyte production and for red blood cell membranes.
• Apparently, women on the pill try to produce extra glutathione, probably to protect themselves against the dangers of peroxidation of fat, as oral contraceptives are known to increase blood lipids and lipoperoxides.
• It is used in an enzyme system which lengthens fatty acid chains.
• It is synergistic with vitamins C and B.

With today's heavily poisoned environment, we therefore need to ensure plenty of cysteine. Reliable data on the cysteine contents of food is not readily available and vegetable sources will, in any case, vary depending on the sulphur level of the soil in which they are grown. Unfortunately, in areas which were glaciated, soil is known to be deficient in sulphur, selenium, iodine and zinc. Red peppers, garlic and eggs are the richest reliable sources of cysteine.

Threonine

Threonine is a little-known essential amino acid. It stimulates the immune system by increasing the weight and activity of the thymus and by increasing antibody production. Our treated food provides us with less threonine than we would get from natural food; for example, wild game birds provide 4 grams per pound, battery chickens only 1 g/lb; white flour does not provide any threonine, wheatgerm provides 1.35g/lb.

Getting a balance

Correct amino acid balance is necessary for many things in the body - for good posture, strong muscles, reproduction, growth, body repair, healthy hair, healthy nails, and so on. But for the immune system, proteins, and hence amino acids, in their right balance are essential:

• To pass on a healthy and efficient immune system to your offspring.

• To make immune cells and weapons, like antibodies, with which to fight.

• To control energy levels. The correct amino acid balance is needed at every stage of digestion, absorption and energy release. We want smooth energy levels all the time, not the high energy peaks followed by low energy troughs which result from too much sugar or refined carbohydrates and too little protein; the latter condition resembles a learner driver in first gear who has not yet worked out how to balance the clutch with the accelerator, and frog-hops down the road.

• To control our moods. Neurotransmitter are body chemicals that make us hungry, thirsty, sexy, aggressive, angry, energetic, depressed, unhappy, etc. They control our moods and emotions, as well as our ability to learn, remember and think. Getting the amino acids right will not make anyone into a genius, but it will allow everyone to reach their full potential.

• Brain chemistry is more dependent on diet than you might think, and can be shown to alter, depending on what is eaten at the last meal: tyrosine is vital in regulating emotional moods; phenylalanine is necessary for adrenaline production and stored fat metabolism; tryptophan increases serotonin in the brain and so may relieve sleeplessness and depression; glutamine improves concentration.

• Unbalanced protein intake can increase the production of uric acid, which can lead to gout.

Many people find that when their amino acid balance is restored, they do not crave junk foods. In contrast, it is perfectly possible to live healthily and well on a vegetarian or vegan diet, although people who do so should make sure that they know how to combine amino acids; it is necessary for a range of incomplete proteins to be eaten at the same meal in order to make complete proteins in the body. In my opinion, it is not possible to live healthily and well on an entirely junk food diet, and people on this sort of diet should not only think seriously about the protein content of their food but about most of the other nutrients as well. Is a passing fancy now worth risking your future health?

Carbohydrates

Carbohydrates make up the greater part of our diet and are obtained from grains, fruit, vegetables, legumes, nuts and most processed foods.

Complex carbohydrates are much the best way to obtain these, as they come complete with the nutrients necessary for their utilisation. They are a bit like time-release capsules. Simple sugars and refined carbohydrates flood the system with sugars as soon as they are absorbed; this provides a quick flash of energy, but it is followed by a long period of lethargy. In contrast, complex carbohydrates release their sugars slowly so that the level of sugar in the blood remains roughly within a normal range, instead of going up and down like a seesaw. An average blood sugar level is around 90 milligrams/100 ml of blood. If this is maintained, energy levels are good. When it gets down to 70 mg/100 ml the biochemistry alters to tell us that we are hungry - amino acid communication. At 65 mg/100 we crave sweets and become easily irritated, moody and uncooperative. If sufficient and appropriate food is eaten, we feel fine, think quickly and clearly, lose our hunger pangs and even find sweets distasteful.

Starch

Starch is the fundamental carbohydrate we consume, and can be obtained from grains, bread, pulses and vegetables like potato.

We should try to be a little more adventurous with our grains. Although we appear to have a wide variety of foods, our national addiction is definitely wheat. Pastas, pizzas, pastries, biscuits, pies, bread and cakes are all apparently different foods when seen on the menu, but in reality are all wheat. Even breakfast cereals 'specialise' in wheat.

Because of this, our immune system views our 'varied' diet as monotonous. It likes a change, so that it does not get fed up with wheat and does not start attacking it. Try barley, rye, rice, corn (maize) and millet sometimes. Choose wholegrain breakfast cereals rather than sugar - and salt-laden refined ones, and eat lots of vegetables, both raw and cooked.

It is a good habit to eat a few raw vegetables as a starter before a cooked meal. This helps your immune system to deal with the following food without having such a fight. It used to be thought that digestive leucocytosis, i.e. migration of white blood cells to the gut wall and their subsequent destruction, occurred whenever and whatever we ate, but it has now been found that this migration of white blood cells to the gut and their destruction only occurs when we eat cooked food. Raw food does not waste immune soldiers, and raw food before a cooked meal lessens the overall destruction of white blood cells.

Just as starch is the carbohydrate storage compound in plants, so glycogen is the carbohydrate storage compound in animals (including humans). But we get very little glycogen in our diet as it is broken down to glucose after the death of an animal. Meat therefore contains sugar. It is especially important for those involved in a lot of physical activity to eat complex carbohydrate, which is then stored as glycogen and can be used for physical energy when required.

Sugars

We need sugars, glucose is the final breakdown product of all carbohydrate and it is what we, and especially our brains,need as a food. But sugars have got a bad name, mainly because our intake is again out of balance with our needs. At present, one-third of our intake of carbohydrate in the United Kingdom is in the form of sucrose - the sugar we buy in the shops. This 'food' provides nothing except energy, and gets stored as saturated fat if it is not used. Much of it is hidden in highly processed foods and drinks, invisible but actively destructive. As we eat nearly 60 per cent of our calories as carbohydrates, we must be eating nearly 20 per cent of our total calorie intake in the form of sucrose. At least, some people are. In fact, some must be eating more than a fifth of their diet as sucrose, to make up for those of us who avoid it as much as possible.

Sucrose is not only nutrient free; it actually requires nutrients for its metabolism, so it has to steal them from somewhere else. It is one of the reasons why vitamin B deficiency is so common. We waste precious nutrients including the B vitamins trying to process this useless sugar. Although sugar is less alien to the immune system than artificial sweeteners, the problem is that we are eating too much of it. Small amounts are fine; but one-fifth of our daily diet is excessive.

Carbohydrates make up the bulk of plant material, and constitute anything from 40 per cent (affluent people) to 90 per cent (poor and protein-deficient people) of our diet. The optimum intake is probably somewhere around 50-60 per cent, preferably consumed in its natural form, complete with fibre and nutrients.

Fibre

Fibre is calorie free and good for slimming as it passes through the system without being digested; it fills you up without giving you anything with which to form fat. But a high-fibre diet does not mean sprinkling bran on everything; in fact, this habit can cause more problems than it solves. Remember that wheat bran is a refined food, just like white flour; whole foods are a better way to take fibre. Oat and rice bran are better.

Dry cereal like cereal fibre goes in at one end and comes out at the other, and does a scouring job in between. If it is taken regularly, preferably as a whole grain, it reduces the build-up of faecal material, and so helps the absorption of nutrients through the intestine. A lifetime on a low-fibre diet will create a much thicker faecal build-up in the intestines, and so absorption of nutrients will be less. Minerals, however, do tend to be attracted to fibre, so eating added fibre with every meal can actually deprive you of minerals. This is another good example of the need to get the balance right.

There are many types of fibre. Gums, resins and pectins, as well as cellulose, which is the major component of plant cell walls, all provide fibre. Ruminant animals can break cellulose down into sugar, but we cannot do this. However, the bugs in our gut do need it in order to stay healthy. So eating greens keeps our welcome guests happy and, in return, they keep us clean and tidy inside and provide us with a bonus of B vitamins, essential amino acids and fats. What a bargain.

A clean gut is obviously better for the immune system. If we are repeatedly constipated, there is a build-up of toxins which can be absorbed into the bloodstream; the immune system has to deal with this. And no self-respecting bugs want to live in a constipated gut. They move out and make room for the less reputable varieties, like candida, who are willing to slum it in these unhealthy living conditions.

22

NATURE'S PHARMACY

There is a growing tendency to reconsider the use of plants and their extracts, which were man's most ancient therapeutic aids. We still rely heavily on them for medicinal drugs, extracting the active ingredients and using these as 'starter kits'. For example, aspirin, digitalis and morphine, to name the obvious few.

Justus von Liebig, a nineteenth century chemist, introduced the concept of metabolism, ie. organisms are alive because of the many chemical reactions that take place in their cells, both building up (anabolism) and breaking down (catabolism). He worked on morphine from the opium poppy, strychnine from Strychnos nux-vomica and quinine from Cinchona bark.

Today, there are a few plant chemicals which are being tested for their potential immunostimulating or healing properties. These are some of the alkaloids, phenols, quinones and terpenes. The opium poppy contains 25 different, known alkaloids of which morphine is the strongest pain reliever (analgesic).

Ancient man knew which plants could be used as food and which were poison, which were best for fuels and dyes, which could be used as drinks and which could be fermented to produce alcoholic beverages, (these were very important then, not only because of the intoxicating effect but because they didn't have modern preservatives and so it was one of the few ways of giving drinks that longer shelf life to last until the next season). He also knew which plants could be used as medicines and which caused hallucinatory, psychedelic and narcotic effects. The trend today is to relearn some of the old remedies, many of which stand up to laboratory investigations.

As many as half of the Earth's species live in the tropical rain forests, which cover less than 2% of the globe. Because of their continued destruction, 20% of these are likely to be extinct by the turn of the century and with them some of the most potent medicines.

Uncaria tomentosa (cat's claw)

Cat's claw, (so called because its thorn is shaped like the claw of a cat), is one of these special plants. It is a woody vine that can grow to over 100 feet in its attempt to reach light in the Peruvian rain forests where it is found, by winding its way up through the trees. The native Indians have long used the root bark of this plant to cure tumours, joint problems and a whole host of other diseases.

Research is in its infancy at present, but so convincing have been the results of some initial trials that the plant has become an endangered species and the Peruvian government has passed legislation to prevent the harvesting and use of the root of either of the two main species (U. tomentosa and U. guianensis). It appears that the bark contains most or all of the medicinal properties and the bark will grow back whereas cutting or damaging the whole root causes death of the entire plant. It is still feared that world-wide demand for this bark is in excess of what can be produced and so, as with ginseng, the purchaser needs to be aware of non-therapeutic substitutes.

All of the research papers I have come across so far have been Austrian, Italian, Hungarian or Chinese in origin. Six oxindole alkaloids were extracted from the root (in 1989, before legislation to prevent use of root). Four of these, isopteropodine, pteropodine, isomitraphylline and isorynchophylline, were shown to increase the ability of white blood cells to carry out phagocytosis, ie. to engulf, digest and so destroy an invading germ. A fifth alkaloid, rynchophylline, studied at the Shanghai College of Traditional Chinese Medicine was shown to have the ability to inhibit platelet aggregation, one of the main problems causing thrombosis, and so possibly useful in preventing thrombosis or strokes.

It has also been shown to contain other potentially useful chemicals such as proanthocyanidins, polyphenols and other plant sterols which reduce inflammation. It is potentially a super-plant with immune-stimulating, antioxidant, anti-inflammatory, anti-tumour and antimicrobial properties.

Austrian researchers have also identified triterpenes as well as additional alkaloids, mitraphylline, isomitraphylline, speciophylline and uncarine F. They have been using these extracts to treat cancer and viral infections. One problem they have come across is that different samples have different amounts of these therapeutic chemicals in, which makes dosage difficult to calculate. It is not yet known whether this is due to location, seasonal or species variation. These researchers also found that the root bark extracts increased the phagocytic activity of the macrophages and polymorphonuclear neutrophiles in vitro, therefore its immunostimulating effect is reasonably certain. They have also isolated some of the alkaloids from the leaves and stalk which could be very useful considering the size of the plant, as far as yield is concerned, although the content of the stalk was small in comparison to the leaf and root bark.

It remains to be seen whether extracts of cat's claw will be the basis of a wonder drug of the future.

Other medicinal plants

Pharmacology is the study of how the functions of living organisms can be modified by chemical substances. In this chapter we are concerned with the chemical substances found in plants. Some plants are poisonous, ie. they contain chemicals which disrupt normal function. Others are medicinal plants which contain chemicals which either promote normal activity or inhibit abnormal activity. Sometimes there is a very fine line between the amount which is therapeutic and that which is toxic. Just because something is natural, doesn't mean that it is necessarily good for you.

We will just consider a few plants which affect the heart and circulatory system as examples of plant magic. Herbalists will know of hundreds of such plants and remedies, but to list them all would take a book in itself and is outside the scope of this book. Suffice here to show examples of plants with healing powers and to demonstrate their potential in the future. Plant remedies have been used for centuries, but were based on trial and error and tended to be lost or classified as 'old wives tales'. We now know that many of them have their roots in scientific fact and they are becoming more and more tried, tested and used.

Leaf of foxglove, (Digitalis purpurea & Digitalis lanata) contains various complex steroidal substances, eg. cardiotonic glycosides such as digitoxin and digoxin. D. lanata has 63 different, known steroidal glycosides! Millions of people are being treated with it or its derivatives for heart problems. Dose is very important as the therapeutic dose is very near to that of the toxic dose.

Glycoside-like compounds are also found in the Liliaceae family and may be used for the treatment of arrhythmias (lack of regular heart beat). Quinidine, an alkaloid isomer of the antimalarial compound, quinine, from the Chinchona tree, may be used similarly.

Diuretics are often used and these remove salt as well as water from the body. Ripe fruit of Juniper (Juniperus communis) contains a volatile oil and resins which act on the kidneys, but this is sometimes too strong and extracts from wild carrot (Daucus carota) or dandelion (Taraxacum officinale) are sometimes used instead. Dandelion is very good because, as a bonus, it contains high levels of potassium which can replace that lost in the urine. (The average diet these days contains a great excess of sodium and a deficiency of potassium which should, ideally, be in balance.)

Tropical plants, bananas, coconuts etc. all contain a lot of potassium. It is well known that more salt is needed in hot climates. However, we err if we just take salt (sodium chloride) tablets, as potassium is just as important and often in short supply.

The root of the shrub Rauvolfia serpentina contains the alkaloid, reserpine which has an effect on noradrenaline, a neurotransmitter which is required for transmission of impulses in turn causing relaxation of smooth muscle in blood vessels and so reducing blood pressure.

Flavonoids in hawthorn (Crataegus monogyra) are used for the treatment of angina, atherosclerosis and thrombosis. Examples of alkaloids with cardioactive properties are sparteine from Broom (Sarothamnus scoparius) which raises blood pressure and one from Motherwort (Leonurus cardiaca), which lowers blood pressure.

Plant magic

We rely heavily on plants, indeed without them we could not survive at all. They provide us with:

1 Utilisable carbon compounds

All of life on earth is ultimately dependent on energy from the sun, however, humans cannot harness this energy directly. We need plants to convert the sun's light energy into chemical energy so that we can use it. They do this by the process of photosynthesis, they take in water and carbon dioxide (our waste product) and using the sun's light energy, make glucose (the basic building block of life which can then be further built up into starches or converted into proteins and fats) and oxygen.

$$6H_2O \quad + \quad 6CO_2 \quad \xrightarrow{\text{light energy from the sun}} \quad C_6H_{12}O_6 \quad + \quad 6O_2$$

water   carbon dioxide   glucose   oxygen

All of the food we eat has come directly or indirectly from plants (eg. if we eat meat from the cow it, in turn, has fed on grass in order to produce its muscle tissue).

2 Oxygen

The waste product of photosynthesis is oxygen. Plants, by their method of feeding, restore the atmosphere's oxygen. This is a very good reason why we should stop destroying the tropical rainforests which produce a great deal of the world's atmospheric oxygen, and should plant trees, parks and gardens in urban areas. The more plants you have in your own personal space, in your home and garden, the better the quality of air around you. Spider plants are excellent indoor plants, renowned for taking in domestic pollutants, purifying the air and requiring very little attention in return. When people say that they talk to their plants and they grow better, it's probably true, not because they can hear them, (biologically they have no mechanism for hearing), but because whilst talking to the plant, you would be breathing out carbon dioxide all over it, giving it a good supplement of one of the raw materials needed for photosynthesis and hence for growth.

3 Medicines

Plants are great restorers of natural balance, whether it be taking in air pollutants and giving out oxygen, converting light energy into utilisable chemical energy, or containing the chemicals necessary to restore biochemical balance once it has been lost. Is it any wonder that they hold the key for healing and restoring normality at all levels? What we need to do is to use each plant's key to open its box and find out what is within. Some plants will be like Pandora's box and contain substances poisonous to us, although they may have a different biological role to fulfil. (Pandora, according to Greek mythology was the first woman on earth, she was given a box that she was ordered never to open but, unable to contain her curiosity, she disobeyed, so releasing all of the evils that plague humanity, the only thing that remained when she closed the box was hope!) Others will contain chemicals that will help us to relieve or cure one ailment or another. We live our lives in the world's garden, it may not be Eden but it provides our food, our water and our air; it contains plants which are our food, those which we must not eat and others which contain some of the secrets of the tree of life, if only we could find them and harness their powers.

Feeling better naturally

Cosmetic uses of natural substances.

• **Almond.** Moisturiser. Oil used to soften and moisturise skin and to eliminate dry or scaly patches. Ground almond, used as a scrub to prevent blackheads, spots and enlarged pores.

• **Angelica.** Odour eliminator. Leaves used in baths, especially foot baths. Root when chewed, freshens breath, removes odour.

• **Apple.** Germicidal. Scent and antibacterial action make it an active ingredient of many hair, skin and hand preparations.

• **Apricot.** Very beneficial for the skin due to its high beta-carotene and polyunsaturated oil content. Used in antiwrinkle preparations, and to prevent stretch marks and signs of ageing necks.

• **Avocado.** Very rich in oils which penetrates the skin well; has healing as well as moisturising properties. Can be used on hair as well as the skin.

• **Banana.** Can be used as a skin cleanser, as can avocado.

• **Bay**. Antiseptic properties. Leaves used in baths and for making perfume.

• **Beer.** Excellent hair rinse, giving good shine.

• **Bicarbonate of soda.** Good cleanser; can be used in toothpastes.

• **Blackberry.** Astringent properties in fruit. Leaves soothe burns.

• **Bran.** As you might expect, bran is used as a abrasive scrub. It can also be used to remove grease and dirt from hair or skin.

• **Camomile.** Highlights white or blonde hair. Also a relaxant in a bath.

• **Carrot.** Juice has long been reputed to benefit skin, hair and eyes when taken internally. Has a mild, light tanning effect when applied topically.

• **Castor oil.** Nail strengthener applied topically.

• **Cinnamon.** Breath freshener. Can also be incorporated into home made toothpaste.

• **Cloves.** Antiseptic and very characteristic smell. Good in baths or as mouth and breath freshener.

• **Cocoa butter.** Useful as a lip gloss.

• **Coconut.** Oil is used as a moisturiser; especially good for sore lips as it is edible. Can use it for cleansing, (commercially used in soaps) and as a suntan oil. It is a saturated oil.

• **Comfrey.** Healing properties. Good for chapped skin and as a bath soak.

• **Corn.** The starch is used as a dry shampoo. The oil, if it is cold pressed (not had the vitamin E taken out and an artificial antioxidant added) is good rubbed into the skin to soften it. Best rubbed in before a bath; then soak in warm water, allowing the oil to penetrate; towel dry. Leaves the skin supple and shiny.

• **Cream.** Good for smooth skin, especially for moisturising around the eyes, which is a particularly sensitive area.

• **Cucumber.** Astringent, but very mild; suitable for sensitive skins. Valuable as a skin cooler after sunbathing, to soothe sore eyes, and as a skin cleanser, helping to prevent blackheads and spots.

• **Dandelion.** Good cleanser; sometimes used in baths, for cleansing properties rather than scent.

• **Eggs.** Egg white 'stretch' the skin, so are good for keeping skin as wrinkle free as possible for its age. Yolks are moisturisers and can be rubbed into the face and hands. Egg as a shampoo gives hair body and shine.

• **Elderflower.** General skin-texture improver.

• **Fennel.** Soothes swollen and sore eyes.

• **Garlic.** Antiseptic. Also stimulates hair growth.

• **Grapefruit.** Good in skin treatments, softening elbows, knees etc. Because it's acidic, like lemon, it is good in bath water or for a hair rinse. The skin and hair should be slightly acidic, and citric fruits are good for restoring this mild acidity after washing, especially if soap has been used. Beware of using concentrated lemon juice on dark hair, if left on it can lighten it considerably and this may not be the effect you want.

• **Honey.** A very effective softener with good healing properties. Good for spotty skins or rough, weather-damaged skins when applied topically. It is antibacterial.

• **Horseradish.** Good for all skin blemishes. Extracts from the root will help to lighten age spots or freckles in some cases. It whitens nails. It does tend to dry the skin if used too often.

• **Lavender.** Often added to any preparation to provide a scent. Cleansing action.

• **Lemon.** Astringent. Like grapefruit, it restores the skin or hair's natural acid balance. It is a good all round addition, also providing vitamin C.

• **Lettuce.** Cleanser and natural, mild tranquilliser.

• **Lime.** Flowers lighten the skin; have a calming effect in the bath.

• **Marigold.** Skin tonic. Also highlights red brown hair.

• **Melon.** Cleanser; moisturiser.

• **Milk**, often used to soften skin - queens used to bathe in it.

• **Myrrh.** Used as a treatment for mouth ulcers. Also in toothpastes, mouth rinses and skin toners. It was used to preserve mummies, so has presertive properties!

• **Nettles.** Used for tired feet and for strengthening hair.

• **Oats.** Used as a scrub for cleansing; also to whiten hands.

• **Olive.** Absorbs the sun's UV rays, so useful as a sunscreen oil. Good for brittle nails or hair.

• **Orange.** Another citrus fruit with an appealing smell.

• **Orris.** Root is good for keeping teeth white, and as a dry shampoo.

• **Parsley.** Valuable as an antidandruff agent, hair rinse for dark hair and to control acne.

• **Peach.** Moisturiser for tired skins.

• **Peppermint.** Used in cosmetics for taste and smell; general use.

• **Pine.** Fragrance is often desired; good in baths.

• **Potato.** Reduces swelling and inflammation, especially for skin and eyes after sunbathing.

• **Rhubarb.** Reddish temporary hair dye.

• **Rose.** Used a lot for scent, but also good for chapped skin.

• **Rosemary.** Especially good for shiny hair and to prevent dandruff. Also can be used in baths, etc, for its scent.

• **Safflower oil.** Even higher in polyunsaturates than sunflower oil; good for body massage.

• **Sage.** Used to whiten teeth and strengthen gums. Stimulant when used on the scalp. Can be used in mouthwashes, toothpastes, etc. because of its scent and taste.

- **Salt.** Antibacterial; helps to heal broken skin, although it can cause severe stinging when initially added. Salt water is very useful for very minor cuts and grazes.
- **Sesame oil.** Also tends to absorb harmful rays from the sun whilst allowing the tanning process, therefore useful as a sunscreen.
- **Strawberry.** Good for alleviating sunburn and whitening teeth. Also good for the skin.
- **Sunflower.** Oil is good for body massage, especially mixed with a scented oil, eg. rose.
- **Tea.** The tannin in tea, whilst not desirable in great quantities internally, is very good for absorbing the sun's more damaging radiation; It is therefore a useful sunscreen (although it washes off in sea or pool/bath). Slightly dyes the skin, so helping you to look tanned. It is sometimes used to brighten dull dark hair and to relieve eye strain.
- **Thyme.** Bath additive and a shampoo.
- **Tomato.** Supposed to reduce the effects of large pores.
- **Vinegar.** Good as a hair rinse to make hair shine (dilute, of course, or it will also make it smell)!
- **Yoghurt.** Like milk, it is good for skin preparations; also as a hair conditioner. It has antifungal properties.

Cosmetics should make us smell good, feel good, look good and do no harm.

Plant magic, medical miracles and body perfect

Modern living and its technology has caused many imbalances in our lives, from our method of movement to the pollution of water and air and the quality of our food. Many of these changes are welcome and beneficial but equally many have undesirable side-effects and cause deleterious, immunological reactions. To every action there is an equal and opposite reaction. This is a basic law for all life, known as the law of Karma. We often try to ignore its wider application by filing it away in the physical sciences as Newton's 3rd law of motion. We need to correct some of these imbalances if we are to minimise premature ageing, degenerative disease and unnecessary illness. There is no doubt that balance is the key to all aspects of life, too much is not always better and too little is never enough.

It is difficult to convince apparently healthy, symptom free people to change the lifestyle and diet that they enjoy, but we are piling more and more nutrient free, chemically laden rubbish into ourselves and expect the immune system to sort it all out and to deal with it. It is possible to change habits gradually and to be just as happy with the healthier habits. Most of us could do with eating less. Words written in an Egyptian pyramid 5,000 years ago still apply today, they are, "Man lives on one quarter of what he eats, his doctor lives on the other three quarters".

A lot of time and money is spent on dress, appearance and external hygiene, but we often ignore the state of the body within. It's necessary to have a 'keep body internally clean and tidy' campaign from time to time.

It is also wise to use 'plant magic' and other natural therapies sometimes, as well as conventional medicine when necessary; they are not mutually exclusive. Each has its own strengths and limitations but may often be used effectively side by side.

Most of all, listen to your own body. It is well equipped with an efficient immune system which is able to resist disease and heal injury if we give it what it needs to do so. If a disease takes hold, our natural instinct is to strengthen our defences to beat the enemy. Our immune system can be our strength or our Achilles heel as it is often one of the first systems to deteriorate if it is not looked after properly. Splash out on pampering your immune system, encourage it but don't let it become overworked and confused so that it starts making mistakes. There is no doubt that the immune system is affected by our diet, lifestyle, thoughts, movements and environment. The good news is that by taking care of and improving these things, we can improve our health. True wealth is what we are, not what we have and we each have control over the type of person we become. No one is guaranteed health and happiness. Life just gives us time and space, (body space). It's up to us to fill it with health, joy and meaning.

USEFUL ADDRESSES

Institute for Optimum Nutrition
Blades Court, Deodar Road, London SW15 2NU   Tel: 0181 877 9993
ION offers courses and consultations with nutrition consultants, plus a national directory of nutrition consultants (see page 159).

Laboratory tests are available for all the tests mentioned in this book, through qualified nutrition consultants. Leading laboratories include Biolab Medical Unit (doctors only) Tel: 0171 636 5959; Immuno Laboratories for IgG ELISA allergy testing Tel: 01435 882 880; and also Larkhall Laboratories Tel: 0181 874 1130.

RECOMMENDED READING

Optimum Nutrition
Patrick Holford, ION Press, 1994. This book defines optimum nutrition and how to achieve it. It contains a step-by-step plan to work out your own diet and supplement programme.

Optimum Nutrition Workbook
Patrick Holford, ION Press, 1995. This 209 page, large format book is packed with informative diagrams and covers all the facts about nutrition and is the sequel to *Optimum Nutrition*.

Dr Braly's Food Allergy and Nutrition Revolution
Dr James Braly, Keats Publishing, 1992. A great 'self-help' book explaining the importance of optimum nutrition in relation to a new way of understanding allergies, explaining why modern day diets have led to increased allergic sensitivity and digestive disorders - and how to get back to health. Very comprehensive.

These books are available from the ION Bookclub, Blades Court, Deodar Road, London SW15 2NU. Please call 0181-871-4576 for a current price list.

INDEX

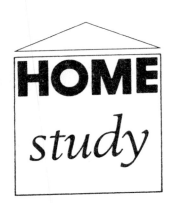

Your car comes with a manual, but what about your body?

What makes you tick? How do you make energy from food? Why do some people age faster - and how can you age more slowly? What's the secret for super-health?

You'll find many answers in **ION's Homestudy Course** (that comes with 3 workbooks, 3 hours of videos, 12 taped lectures and step by step instructions to give you a solid grounding in 10 weeks). You'll learn more than you thought possible and have fun doing it with practical homework and experiments.

Part 1 HOW YOUR BODY WORKS teaches you how to improve digestion and absorption, balance nerves and hormones, and boost immune power. The second part **FOOD & NUTRITION**, looks at everything from the politics of food to wholefood cookery. You'll find out how to prevent heart disease and protect against cancer and arthritis, as well as learning how to detect your own food intolerances. In the final part, **INDIVIDUAL NUTRITION**, you'll learn how to work out individually tailored programmes. You'll find out all about nutrition for children and the elderly, including nutritional 'first aid'.

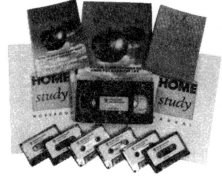

By the end of the course you'll know enough to keep yourself and your family healthy. When you enrol you'll get all the course materials, plus your own 'telephone tutor' to help you with any questions you have. Anyone can do it. All you need is a keen interest in nutrition.

Price: £150   **Members price: £135**

I O N

The Institute for Optimum Nutrition is a non profit-making independent organisation that exists to help you promote your health through nutrition. ION was founded in 1984 and is based in London. ION offers educational courses starting with a one-day introductory course right up to a three year training to become a nutrition consultant; a clinic for one-to-one consultations; publications and ION's magazine, Optimum Nutrition, which goes out free to members. If you'd like to receive more details please complete the details below.

Please send me your:

☐   FREE Information Pack on all ION services
☐   FREE BookClub Bulletin
☐   Directory of Nutrition Consultants
       (enclose £2 plus A5 SAE)

I'd like to order the following books: *(please list title, quantity & price)*

_____

_____

_____

I enclose £ _____ payable to ION (Please add 10% for p&p)

First Name: _____ Surname: _____

Address: _____

_____ Postcode: _____

Now send this to: ION, Blades Court, Deodar Road,
London SW15 2NU (Tel: 0181 877 9993)